SHIATS

GW01003671

After obtaining a degree in zoology and teaching biology in schools and colleges, Oliver Cowmeadow encountered Eastern philosophy and medicine in 1980. Immediately taken by the Oriental view of life and health, he intensively studied the Eastern philosophy and its application in Shiatsu and macrobiotics in London, Boston and on the Continent.

Oliver moved to the south west of England to begin practising Shiatsu, and in 1985 founded the Devon School of Shiatsu, one of the first schools in the UK offering a full training in Shiatsu. He has played a significant part in the development of the Shiatsu Society, the professional body representing Shiatsu in the UK, especially in the areas of curriculum development and training standards. This is his fifth book on the Eastern approach to health.

Oliver Cowmeadow

SHIATSU

A PRACTICAL INTRODUCTION

INDEX COMPILED BY LYN GREENWOOD

SAFFRON WALDEN
THE C.W. DANIEL COMPANY LIMITED

Originally published by Element Books in 1992
This much revised edition first published in 2002 in the United Kingdom by
The C.W. Daniel Company Limited
1 Church Path, Saffron Walden,
Essex CB10 1JP, United Kingdom

© Oliver Cowmeadow 2002

ISBN 0 85207 359 3

Produced in association with
Book Production Consultants plc,
25-27 High Street, Chesterton, Cambridge, CB4 1ND.
Designed by Marion Hughston.
Printed and bound in the United Kingdom by
St Edmundsbury Press Ltd, Bury St Edmunds, Suffolk.

CONTENTS

PREFACE

This book has a dual purpose. Firstly it intends to introduce a different way of seeing the world and ourselves, based on the Energetic nature of life. While many traditional cultures have recognised the Energetic basis of life and health, modern Western culture has almost exclusively focused on the material aspect. Gaining a perception and knowledge of the human Energetic make-up opens up new possibilities for understanding our health and how to alleviate health problems.

Secondly this book gives a comprehensive guide for the beginner to learn the healing art of Shiatsu, a system of healing that primarily works on an Energetic level. It is a practical method of learning to perceive the Energetic nature of the human body and being, and to use Energy to promote health and alleviate sickness.

Although the roots of Shiatsu are very old, it developed a great deal in the twentieth century, gaining from the contributions of a number of different sources of wisdom. While based on traditional Chinese medicine, this century it has been enriched and extended by modern Shiatsu teachers like Toru Namikoshi and Shizuto Masunaga in Japan and Wataru Ohashi in the West, by the modern Western understanding of anatomy and physiology, and by macrobiotic teachings, which combine a traditional Eastern understanding of life and health with the modern Western scientific understanding.

While everyone giving Shiatsu is using the same basic ideas and technique, the variety of sources of knowledge and techniques used in Shiatsu has created a number of different styles. This book represents my particular style drawn from traditional Shiatsu teachings, macrobiotics, and other sources on the nature of our subtle Energetic being. It will give a sound foundation in understanding and giving Shiatsu, and can be used as a basis for further study in any style you may later encounter.

HOW TO USE
THIS BOOK

The format of this book is based on the many Introductory Shiatsu Classes that I have taught in Devon and Cornwall. It is designed as a step-by-step guide, to be read and used in sequence chapter by chapter. Part 1 gives an introduction to the approach of Shiatsu and our Energetic make-up. This section can be quite quickly read through and the exercises to perceive Energy practised.

The chapters of Part 2 are practical in nature, and give instruction in learning to give Shiatsu. After first working through these chapters you may want to read no further, and keep using this section over a few weeks to perfect your learning to give an effective full-body Shiatsu treatment.

Part 3 contains chapters that will give you a lot of extra information to experiment with for months to come. While you might be drawn to reading through them earlier on, each one primarily gives information to be practically applied in your giving of Shiatsu and in your daily life. As such they will take time to digest and assimilate.

Bon appetit!

◆ A Note on Nomenclature

In this book some words begin with a capital letter, to show that they are being used to represent an Oriental concept. For example 'Energy' refers to the Oriental idea of subtle Energy which is different from the usual Western idea of 'energy', and 'Kidneys' refers to an Oriental concept which is different from the Western scientific understanding of the kidneys as physical organs. These Oriental concepts will be explained in the text of the book, but you can also refer to the Glossary for brief definitions.

◆ Author's Note

This book is not meant to be used as a substitute for professional medical help. Please consult a doctor or other qualified health practitioner if you are in any doubt about the cause and treatment of any health problem.

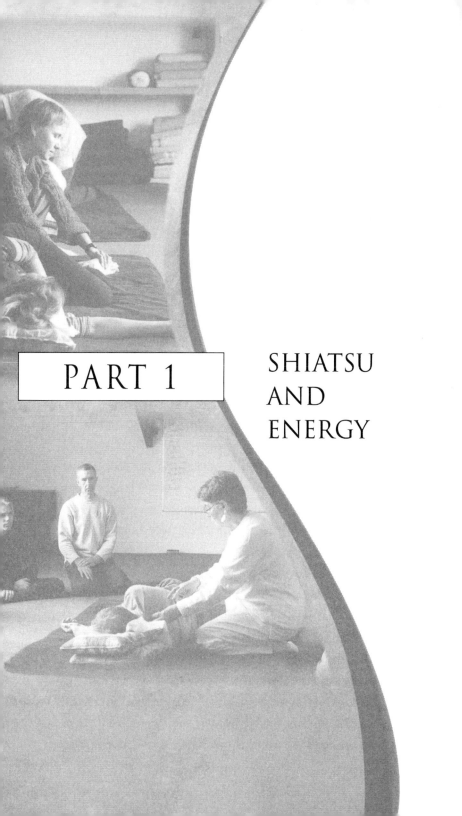

PART 1

SHIATSU
AND
ENERGY

Chapter 1

WHAT IS SHIATSU?

The word 'Shiatsu' is Japanese, and literally means 'finger pressure', as this is the main technique used in giving Shiatsu. Pressure is also applied to the body with the palms of the hands, and sometimes with the elbows, knees and feet to give stronger pressure. Stretching exercises are also applied to increase flexibility in a similar way to yoga or other 'loosening-up' exercises.

Shiatsu could be said to be like a combination of acupuncture and massage. Like the ancient Chinese art of acupuncture, Shiatsu works on the flow of Chi, Ki, or 'Life-Energy' that circulates through the body in specific channels or Meridians. By promoting the steady and unimpeded flow of Ki and rebalancing the flow where it has become either excessive or deficient, health is increased and many health problems alleviated. However, rather than inserting needles into the body, Shiatsu uses touch with the hands or other parts of the body. As with massage, this touch by another human can have great healing effects in itself. We have all put a hand over a knock or other painful part of the body to relieve pain, or have experienced how much the holding of a hand, or an arm around the shoulder, can relieve suffering. Shiatsu is like a specialised system of touching that will have the greatest healing effects.

◆ A Brief History of Shiatsu

The foundation of Shiatsu lies in ancient Chinese medicine. The earliest recorded writing on Chinese medicine, *The Yellow Emperor's Classic of Internal Medicine,* written over two thousand years ago, contains a wealth of information on the causes of many illnesses, and how they may be remedied using changes in diet and lifestyle and with acupuncture and massage. This ancient Oriental medicine has been greatly enlarged and developed over the last two thousand years. This form of massage found its way to Japan, and was called Anma. Anma was often practised by blind people, and was widely used to treat common ailments.

During the twentieth century in Japan, new influences on Anma from both the traditions of the East and modern Western science shaped it into what is now called Shiatsu. In the 1970s, Shiatsu began spreading to the West where it has caught on with amazing rapidity. In Britain early students of Shiatsu have been instrumental in setting up a number of schools offering professional courses in Shiatsu, so that the number of qualified Shiatsu therapists is rapidly increasing. The Shiatsu Society has been established as the professional body promoting Shiatsu and maintaining high standards of practice in the UK. More recently a lot of media coverage has brought the benefits of Shiatsu to the public's attention, and it is gaining wide acceptance as a powerful and effective therapy.

◆ Eastern and Western Medicine

In many ways the philosophical approaches to life and health are opposite in the East and West. This does not necessarily mean that they are in conflict with each other or cannot be used side by side, but rather that they take a very different view of health and sickness. In fact these two opposite approaches complement each other very well, as do all opposites.

One particular opposite viewpoint of these two great efforts to understand health and cure sickness is that modern Western medicine studies the physical or material functioning of the body, such as its mechanical working and chemical nature, whereas traditional Eastern medicine primarily sought to understand the Energetic basis of life, health and disease. This Energy is called Chi in Chinese, Ki in Japanese, and Prana in India, and has been called 'Life Energy', 'Orgone Energy', or 'Subtle Energy' in the West. It is not the same as the Western scientific idea of energy, which is based on the energetic content of physical matter, such as the amount of heat produced by the burning of food measured in calories or joules. Rather it is believed that a more subtle form of Energy pervades the whole universe, and that it is from this universal Energy that matter is formed. Living organisms are seen as particularly active centres of subtle Energy, their very life depending on constant nourishment, not only by physical nutrients but also by this Energy.

So far no scientific instruments have been able directly to detect or measure subtle Energy, although some instruments can detect it indirectly, such as little instruments measuring skin resistance that can be used to find acupuncture points over the body. This Energy can be felt quite easily by other living organisms, and anyone can learn to perceive it for themselves. (The exercises in Chapter 3 will enable you to do so.)

Shiatsu, like acupuncture, affects a particular system of Energy in the body, that of the Meridians. *Meridian* is a French word (acupuncture was first introduced from the East to France) meaning channel, and describes the channels of Energy which flow over the surface of the body and into the interior of the body to the Organs. The surface part of the Meridians offers an easy way to affect the flow of Energy through all of the body through simple touch, or through the insertion of needles as in acupuncture, or through the application of heat as in moxibustion. These efforts to affect Energy flow in the Meridians are often centred on particular points along the

Meridians which have been found to be especially effective. These are known as acupuncture or acupressure points, or as Tsubos in Japanese.

◆ The Role of Shiatsu Today

Shiatsu has two main applications or roles in society today. Firstly as a therapy offered by qualified practitioners who have studied the subject in depth, and secondly by anyone who has studied Shiatsu a little from books or in short courses to relax and deal with minor health problems of family members and friends. Let's look at Shiatsu as a therapy first.

The rapid rise in popularity of Shiatsu would suggest that there is a great need for it at this time. This, indeed, I think is true, one of the main reasons being that it is effective in remedying many problems which the current predominant form of medicine can do little for. For example, many people suffer from problems in which no physical changes can be found in the blood, body chemistry or body structure. Orthodox medicine can therefore offer little or nothing to remedy the problem, except perhaps a palliative to remove the pain or other symptom. Some examples are cases of back pain, headaches, migraines, other aches, pains or chronic tension in the body, insomnia, irregularities in menstrual cycles or painful periods, low libido or vitality, Chronic Fatigue Syndrome (also called ME), and prevalent negative moods like depression, anxiety or worry.

Shiatsu, with its basis of Oriental medicine, has the means to understand how certain definite imbalances in Energy create these kinds of problems, and can therefore often alleviate them. On many occasions I have seen clients who have various 'minor' ailments of this kind, which are nevertheless interfering with their living a normal happy life, and who have been told that physically there is nothing wrong with them. Sometimes the inner feelings of the client are vague, such as feeling weak in the legs, especially when having to stand and talk in front of people, or having an 'empty head' with an inability to think clearly or remember simple things, and the lack of acknowledgement that something is definitely wrong has left them thinking they may be a little mad. In these cases clients are enormously relieved when assured that the symptoms are definitely real and can be perfectly explained by Oriental theory. A single treatment or a series of weekly treatments is very often effective in eradicating these kinds of problem.

Besides giving the actual treatment, most Shiatsu practitioners may also give advice on how clients may themselves do things to help improve their health and alleviate their problems. This may take the form of changes in diet, specific exercises to practise, more regular exercise, or certain changes in a person's lifestyle.

Often when people go to a Shiatsu therapist to remedy a specific problem, over a number of treatments they also experience other benefits, such as sleeping more deeply, feeling calmer, more centred and less uptight, feeling lighter and brighter, or the disappearance of old aches and pains. In fact some people will visit a Shiatsu therapist regularly just for these more general health benefits. This highlights the fact that as well as being an effective remedy for many specific health problems, Shiatsu also promotes overall health of the body, mind and spirit. In this way it acts preventatively, reducing the chances of a person becoming ill in the future.

Shiatsu can also be learnt at a basic level by anyone for their own benefit and for that of their family and friends. At this level there is not the knowledge to help with many of the more serious problems that a qualified Shiatsu therapist may be able to deal with, nevertheless, even after just a little study and practise the benefits to the receiver can be great. After attending an introductory class many of my students have reported helping relieve friends' minor backaches, knee problems, aching shoulders, insomnia and other problems. And then there are the wider benefits of having tension and stress removed from the body, calming the nervous system, increased Energy, and a greater sense of aliveness that comes from a better overall flow of Energy through the Meridians.

◆ Can Anyone Learn to Give Shiatsu?

Yes! You don't have to have any special abilities to be able to learn Shiatsu, and anyone can learn to sense Energy in time. Obviously some people may learn a little more quickly, especially those who have had some experience in massage or other forms of bodywork, or in healing, but virtually anyone can learn to give effective Shiatsu. One advantage of Shiatsu is that it does not require great muscular strength, and is not physically taxing to give. So children, older people or lightly built people can give Shiatsu as effectively as more athletic types.

◆ The Benefits of Learning Shiatsu

Here I would like to report on some of the benefits and joys that learning Shiatsu has brought to myself and my students, and may well bring to you.

1. In learning Shiatsu one learns more about one's own health, and how one can improve it, as well as how to remedy many common problems and help prevent future illness.

2. Shiatsu is such a simple way of healing, just using the hands,

which we carry with us everywhere! So you can offer your healing help at almost any time and in any place. Practically everyone enjoys receiving Shiatsu and benefits from the deep relaxation and healing it brings.

3. In Shiatsu we heal with our caring touch. It is a way of communicating our love and compassion for others in a very direct way. Giving Shiatsu to our family and friends is a wonderful way of nourishing others and strengthening our relationships.

4. Giving Shiatsu is an uplifting experience. By the giving of our Energy, we receive more Energy. When Shiatsu is given in a calm, relaxed and compassionate way, the giver feels physically, mentally and spiritually uplifted and Energized. This contrasts with many activities which tire us by using up our Energy.

5. If you can, learn to give Shiatsu with a friend so that you can practise on each other. You will then receive Shiatsu regularly, which is a great help in your learning of Shiatsu, and also means that you will receive its healing benefits.

6. If you enjoy giving Shiatsu you may well consider practising Shiatsu as a career. Since the introduction of Shiatsu to Britain in the 1970s, there are now schools in many parts of the country training people to give Shiatsu professionally (a list of schools can be obtained from the Shiatsu Society address given at the end of the book). If you discover a strong attraction to this healing art, you may wish to continue to study Shiatsu to reach a professional level.

7. Shiatsu is a potent method of self-development. It has many similarities to some other Eastern methods of personal development such as aikido, tai chi, chi kung, yoga and meditation. In learning Shiatsu one develops many inner qualities that are equally useful in the rest of one's life. These include becoming more centred and grounded and able to stay calm and relaxed while busy or under pressure, developing a greater sensitivity to other people and perceptivity of their health, moods and thoughts, calming of the mind and enhanced intuition.

Usually I give Shiatsu treatments every week. Occasionally I am involved in other work and do not give any for a while. I so miss the unique experience of giving Shiatsu that I end up longing to get my hands on someone, and when I do, I feel so much better! You too may get bitten by the Shiatsu bug and end up an addict. It is my sincere wish that you do.

Chapter 2

OUR ENERGETIC CONSTITUTION

I n giving Shiatsu, we are primarily working with our own and another person's Energy. Those of us brought up in modern Western culture are generally quite unaware of the Energetic nature of life and of all forms and phenomena. In contrast, most developed cultures in past millennia clearly perceived Energy as the basis of life. For example in India it was called 'Prana', in China 'Chi' and in Japan 'Ki'. In the ancient languages of these countries their word for Energy crops up in all kinds of phrases and expressions; it was an integral part of their understanding of their lives and the universe. Yet most languages of modern societies do not even have a word for this Energy. In recent times various words have come into use, such as 'Life Energy', 'Orgone Energy', and 'Vital Energy'. In the rest of this book Ki or simply Energy will be used.

Because Ki is so little recognized in modern, materially orientated culture, you will probably have little or no experience of perceiving it. Don't lose heart! Everyone can learn to perceive Ki, and appreciate how it is an integral part of life. Learning the art of Shiatsu is an excellent way of learning to perceive Ki. With time and practise the world of Ki can become every bit as definite as the physical world. To help you appreciate the world of Ki, it may be helpful to describe briefly the Oriental understanding of the nature of the universe.

The diagram opposite illustrates the relationship between the Physical, Energetic and Spiritual worlds. In the last couple of centuries Western culture has focused on the scientific investigation of the material world, and seeks to explain the nature of life and health in material terms. In contrast, Oriental cultures have looked more at the Energetic world, which is seen as being much larger and encompassing the world of matter. Matter is seen as the most condensed form of Energy, with a continual interchange of Energy condensing to form matter, and matter disintegrating to form Energy. This idea or observation has been demonstrated to some extent by modern physics, which has produced the disintegration of atoms into energy, and the formation of atomic particles by energy.

The modern Western concept of energy is associated with matter, such as the number of calories that some food will produce when fully burnt up. Other forms of energy include various types of electromagnetic energy such as light, X-rays and radio waves. The Eastern concept of Energy is quite distinct from this more physical form of energy. It is of a more subtle nature, that is easily perceived by living organisms such as human beings, but is yet to be measured by a scientific instrument, although this may well happen in the future.

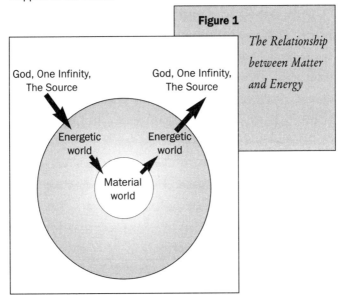

Figure 1

The Relationship between Matter and Energy

God, One Infinity,
The Source

God, One Infinity,
The Source

Energetic world

Energetic world

Material world

And where does Energy come from? The idea of God, One Infinity, The Source, or a state of Absolute Oneness is universal, and has been given different names in different cultures. This state is the source of Energy, matter and life, and at the same time encompasses all Energy, matter and phenomena. The aim of religions and philosophies worldwide has been to raise human consciousness to appreciate God, or the Absolute state. Raising our awareness to appreciate the world of Energy is a step in this direction.

In this traditional view, life is created by Energy. Organized patterns of Energy create an organized physical body, and our emotions, feelings, thoughts and other levels of consciousness are particular manifestations of Energy. When there is abundant Energy, there is aliveness. When energy is weak or absent, there is lifelessness. So if we want to understand life, we need to understand Energy!

In the rest of this chapter we will briefly survey the major systems of Energy that make up our human being, to give a comprehensive idea of our Energetic constitution. In many traditional cultures, people's awareness of Energy was much greater, and they described several major systems of Energy in the human body. As we become more sensitive to Energy, we too can perceive these Energy systems and confirm their presence to ourselves. You may already be familiar with some of them. In particular the Oriental systems of Organs, Meridians and Tsubos which are most used in Shiatsu, will be introduced.

◆ The Subtle Body System

Many teachings from around the world describe a number of subtle Energetic bodies in addition to the physical body, including yoga teachings, vedantic scriptures, theosophical knowledge and Western researches. These subtle Energetic bodies are seen as overlying the physical body, and extending outside the physical boundary of the body to different distances to form the aura. Each is of a different frequency or 'fineness' of Energy, and so maintains its integrity, just as a number of radio or television stations use different frequencies of radio waves, and so do not interfere with each other.

The number of subtle bodies described varies a little, although there is general agreement on the denser Energetic bodies shown in Figure 2 on page 19.

The **ETHERIC BODY** is the densest level of subtle Energy, and is closely associated with the functioning of the physical body. It extends a few inches beyond the skin and it is probably the etheric body that has been detected by Kirlian photography. The Meridian and Organ systems described later probably exist mainly as part of the etheric body. The first two exercises in Chapter 3 will enable you to feel the etheric body around your hands and over another person. Many forms of healing using the hands work on the etheric level.

The **ASTRAL BODY** is of a higher frequency or finer level of subtle Energy than the etheric body, and extends several feet from the physical body. The astral body is the vehicle of our emotions and, to the clairvoyant able to see it, it varies in shape and colour according to the emotions being experienced by a person.

Although the astral aura is more difficult to perceive directly, many daily experiences involve it. Interactions with other people are often primarily on an emotional level, and bring about changes in the astral body. When one spends time with someone expressing strong emotions, one tends to pick up the Energy of those emotions in one's own astral body. After leaving that person one may then continue to feel that emotion for some time. One may pick up on positive emotions like joy, courage or confidence, or negative emotions like doubt, depression or anger. A way to avoid picking up negative emotions is to be mentally conscious of the emotions being given out and to make the mental decision not to take on those emotions. One can then be open and sympathetic without the unfortunate consequence of taking on the other's negative emotions.

When two people meet they generally keep a certain safe distance from each other, maintaining their 'personal space', and to approach too closely feels uncomfortable. Basically they stay just far enough away to avoid their astral bodies overlapping. Once two people feel safe with each other or have some emotional relationship, then the need to keep their astral bodies separated goes, and a hug or other close contact feels comfortable.

The **MENTAL BODY** is composed of yet finer subtle Energy, and extends further out from the physical body. It is the vehicle of the intellect or thinking mind, and contains specific thoughtforms. To the clairvoyant able to perceive the mental aura, ideas and concepts that a person is conveying can be seen like pictures. It is also the medium of telepathy. When the mental body is developed, it allows an individual to think clearly and to focus mental energies with force and clarity.

The physical, etheric, astral and mental bodies together form a person's personality.

The **CAUSAL BODY** is also called the higher self or soul. It is composed of still finer subtle Energy and extends out far beyond the other bodies. It deals more with intuitive perceptions and understanding. Whereas the mental body is concerned more with analysing or dividing things up in order to understand them, the causal body is synthetic or wholistic, understanding the essence of things and their connection with the whole. In the reincarnation theory, it is considered that at death the physical, astral and mental bodies die while the causal body, or soul, continues on to new lives, where it takes on a new personality in order to develop itself further.

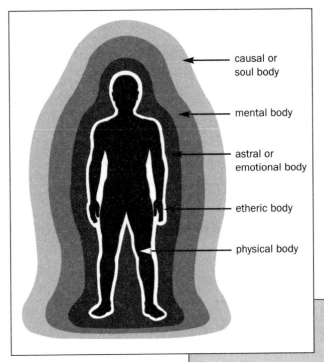

causal or
soul body

mental body

astral or
emotional body

etheric body

physical body

Figure 2

*The Physical and
Energetic Bodies*

In understanding health and healing a few points can be made on the inter-relationships of our various subtle bodies. Firstly, these bodies contain our consciousness on different levels, consciousness of our bodies, emotions, thoughts and intuition. Our consciousness changes levels frequently as we shift our attention between these different levels, and so different bodies are activated. During the process of maturing and personal development, a person's consciousness widens and the higher levels become more active. Whereas a young child is concerned mainly with its physical and emotional experience, in youth the mental faculties become more active, and in a mature adult intellectual and intuitive abilities become more developed.

Secondly, energy passes between the bodies, down to more materialised levels or up to finer levels. Therefore changes in the physical body will affect the etheric body, and through that the emotional, mental and causal bodies. That is to say our physical health is the foundation of health at other levels. Likewise, our emotions or thoughts will have an effect on our physical body and affect our physical health, and events on a causal or soul level will affect all the other bodies or levels of our being.

Thirdly, from the point above it is clear that it is necessary to have a wide variety of healing methods to deal with all the different bodies. Modern scientifically orientated medicine primarily affects the physical body with its use of surgery, chemically based drugs, radiation therapy and so on. Many traditional healing methods primarily act on the etheric body, such as acupuncture and Shiatsu. Other traditional and modern approaches to healing are primarily directed at restoring to health or developing the emotional, mental and causal bodies.

Shiatsu techniques primarily work on the Meridians, which are a part of the etheric body, and through this level bring about changes on a physical, emotional and mental level. However, as an individual becomes more sensitive to Energy on other finer levels, they can also work directly on these.

◆ The Spiritual Channel and Chakras

The strongest flow of Energy in the body is in the spiritual channel or Sushumna, running from the top of the head to the base of the torso. This channel is charged by Energy coming from above and below. When we think of ourselves just as a physical body, it seems that we are quite separate from anything outside of our physical boundary, the skin. When we see ourselves as Energy, this separation disappears. We only exist because of the constant flow of Energy into us from other people, from the earth and other living organisms, from the sun, planets, stars and outer space.

Figure 3

The Spiritual Channel

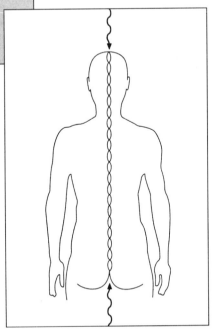

When our body is erect, the flow of these two forces is greatest, increasing the activity of the physical body, the mind and spiritual awareness. Hence if you are reading a demanding book, playing a musical instrument, or doing anything else that demands a great concentration of Energy, it is much easier if one sits up with a straight back rather than slumping or lying down. On the other hand if one wants to relax it is better to lie down. A straight, upright posture has long been recognized as desirable for meditation, and even by school teachers with their sometimes frequent admonishments to 'sit up straight' and 'don't slouch'!

On the spiritual channel there are seven main centres of Energy, often called Chakras. CHAKRA is a Sanskrit word meaning 'wheel', as this is how they can appear to a clairvoyant who can see them. The Chakras are a part of the subtle Energy bodies. Each Chakra has an etheric component, nourishing the surrounding organs and their functions, and also a specific endocrine gland, producing hormones in the body. Each Chakra also has an astral or emotional component, and a mental and causal component, and so forms a centre of consciousness. The main functions of the seven Chakras are summarized in the table below.

Chakra	Gland	Physical organs and parts governed	Emotional, mental and spiritual functions
Crown	Pineal	Upper brain and right eye.	Spiritual awareness, spiritual will-to-be.
Ajna or Brow	Pituitary	Lower brain, left eye, ears, nose, and nervous system.	Higher mind, intuitive perception and understanding.
Throat	Thyroid	Lungs, mouth, throat, vocal cords, shoulders, arms, hands and lymphatic system.	Self-expression, communication, creativity.
Heart	Thymus	Heart, circulatory system, Vagus nerve and breasts.	Love, compassion, service to humanity, awareness of self.
Solar Plexus	Pancreas	Stomach and digestive system, spleen, liver and gall bladder.	Personal power, desire, source of emotions.
Sacral	Gonads	Reproductive system, lower back, legs and feet.	Physical and mental vitality, grounded-ness, sexual energy, relationships and self-esteem.
Base	Adrenals	The spine and skeleton, kidneys, and bladder autonomic nervous system.	Physical will-to-be and procreation.

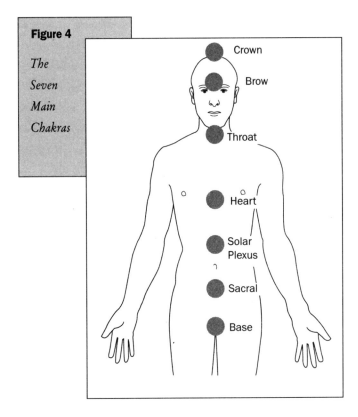

Figure 4

The Seven Main Chakras

Crown

Brow

Throat

Heart

Solar Plexus

Sacral

Base

With the subtle bodies we saw that with the development of consciousness over a lifetime, activity tends to shift to finer bodies, from the physical and etheric to the astral, mental and causal. A similar progression occurs in Chakra activity. While all the Chakras are active in supporting the physical functioning of the body, in emotional, mental and spiritual activity there is a development from the lower Chakras to the upper Chakras. The lowest three Chakras are concerned with our personal survival and our physical and emotional relations with other people and the outside world. The diaphragm can be thought of as a borderline between these 'lower' functions and our 'higher' human functions or qualities. The fourth and fifth

Chakras, the heart and throat, become more active as individuals develop their ability to love and become creative in communicating ideas and concepts. With an increased intuitive understanding of the nature of life and the universe, the sixth, brow Chakra becomes more active. The seventh, crown Chakra only becomes fully active when people have developed far in their awareness, on a spiritual level, of the unity of all life. Thus every change in conciousness is reflected in a change in the activity of the Chakras.

As we saw with the subtle bodies, there is also a movement of Energy between the different subtle bodies within each Chakra. Therefore if there is a change at one level, this will tend to create changes in all the other bodies of the same Chakra. For example, if there is a physical problem, say in the throat, a person often, but not invariably, may also be suffering from a difficulty in expressing his or her inner feelings and thoughts.

◆ The Oriental Concept of Organs

In Oriental medicine the Organs have a wider meaning based on their Energetic functions. For example the Oriental idea of the Kidneys includes not only the physical kidneys and their function of controlling water metabolism, but also the Energetic functions of nourishing the bones, spine and brain, the ears and the hair, and creating willpower and memory. Therefore problems in any of these areas can be due to an imbalance in Kidney Energy.

Twelve main Organs are described in Chinese medicine. Six are concerned with the storage of Energy, and are called Zang. The other six are concerned with *transforming* food and drink into Energy to be stored in the Zang, and with the excretion of waste products. These are called Fu. The Zang all include a 'solid' Organ such as the Liver, whereas the Fu all include a 'hollow' Organ such as the Stomach.

Each of the Zang is paired with a Fu because of a similarity in function. The six pairs are shown in the table below together with their main functions. Note that the physical organ of the Pancreas is generally considered to be included in the Spleen Organ. The Heart Governor and Triple Heater Organs do not have a direct physical counterpart as with the other Organs. The Heart Governor is closely associated with the Heart, and one of its functions is to protect the Heart. The Triple Heater includes the three heaters or burning places where heat and Energy are produced: the chest, solar plexus and the lower abdomen.

ZANG	FU
Lungs • Intake of Ki from air • Combining Ki from air with Ki from food to nourish the whole body • Mental vitality and positivity	**Large Intestine** • Receives food from the Small Intestine, absorbs wanted fluids and excretes unwanted matter in the stools • Ability to 'let go'; self-confidence
Spleen • Transformation of Ki from food into Ki for the body • Gives ability to concentrate, think and analyse	**Stomach** • 'Rots and ripens' food in preparation for extraction of wanted Ki and nutrients by the Spleen, Small and Large Intestines • Nourishes intellectual thinking
Heart • Helps in formation of Blood from the Ki from food and air • Circulates the Blood, and controls the Blood Vessels • Houses the Mind, including our consciousness, thinking, feeling and long-term memory	**Small Intestine** • Receives food from the stomach and separates the nutritious parts from those that are not wanted which are passed on to the large intestine • Mental discrimination and decision-making
Kidneys • Provides fundamental Ki for all other Organs, and for birth, growth, development and reproduction • Nourishes the spine, bones and brain • Gives impetus and willpower	**Bladder** • Stores unwanted fluids and excretes them in the urine • Gives courage

ZANG (Cont)	FU (Cont)
Heart Governor (Pericardium or Heart Protector) • Protects and aids the Heart • Circulation of the Blood around the body • Influences relationships with others	**Triple Heater (Triple Burner)** • Distributes Ki and warmth throughout the body • Opens emotional interactions with other people
Liver • Ensures a smooth flow of Ki to produce optimum physiological functioning and emotional stability • Creates humour, creativity and positive emotions, and the ability to plan	**Gall Bladder** • Stores bile produced by the Liver and secretes it into the Intestines • Ability to make decisions and move forwards into action

◆ The Meridian System

The Energy system most used in Shiatsu is the system of Meridians. Each of the twelve Organs is linked with a Meridian, or channel of Energy, so that we have the Liver Meridian, Heart Meridian, and so on. Part of each Meridian travels through the body, connecting with various Organs and Chakras, and partly over the surface of the body. The Lung Meridian, for example, travels through the lungs and throat, then emerges onto the surface of the body at the front of the shoulder, and travels down the arm to end on the thumb. One end of each of the Meridians is inside the body, and the other end is on the hands feet.

These twelve main Meridians are bilateral; that is there is an identical Meridian on both sides of the body. There are two more Meridians used in Shiatsu: the Governing Vessel that runs up the centre of the back of the body, and the Conception Vessel (or Directing Vessel) that runs up the centre of the front of the body. On each Meridian there are various places which are particularly useful in changing the Energy flow in the whole Meridian. These are often called acupuncture or acupressure points, and in Shiatsu are called Tsubos. The diagrams on pages 28 and 29 show the pathways of the Meridians over the surface of the body.

Energy flows into the Meridians from the Chakras and the Organs of the body, and also from the outside into the ends of the Meridians on the hands and feet, and through the Tsubos. Each Meridian also has a short connecting pathway to two other Meridians, so that Energy flows from one Meridian to another. This Energy flows cyclically through the twelve main Meridians, as shown in Figure 6.

Working on the Meridians has a variety of effects. Firstly, because they run over the body surface and also into the body, working on the outside of the body affects the internal functioning of the Organs. The basic Shiatsu treatment that you will learn to give in Chapter 6 will help improve the Organ functioning, as well as have a beneficial effect on the hormonal system and the autonomic nervous system (that controls many body functions that automatically happen, such as movements of the intestines and bladder). With further training in Shiatsu, treatments can help alleviate a wide range of problems within the body. How amazing to be able to help the inside of the body by working simply with your hands on the outside of the body!

Secondly, the flow of Energy in the Meridians over the surface of the body affects the muscles and joints. Therefore many problems on the body surface can be aided with Shiatsu, such as headaches, tension in muscles, and backaches. Shiatsu is one of the most effective remedies for many of these kinds of problems.

Thirdly, the flow of Energy through the Meridians also affects our moods, emotions and thinking. So Shiatsu often helps lift

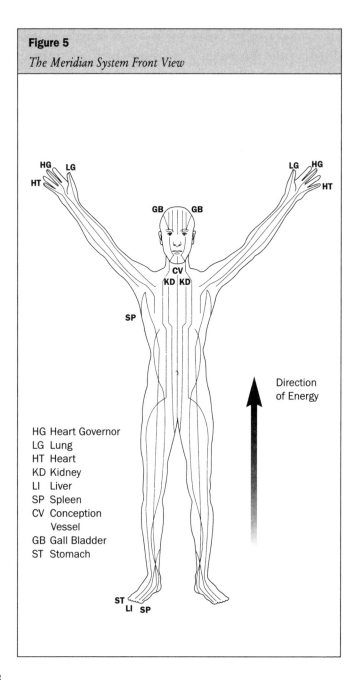

Figure 5

The Meridian System Front View

HG Heart Governor
LG Lung
HT Heart
KD Kidney
LI Liver
SP Spleen
CV Conception
     Vessel
GB Gall Bladder
ST Stomach

Direction of Energy

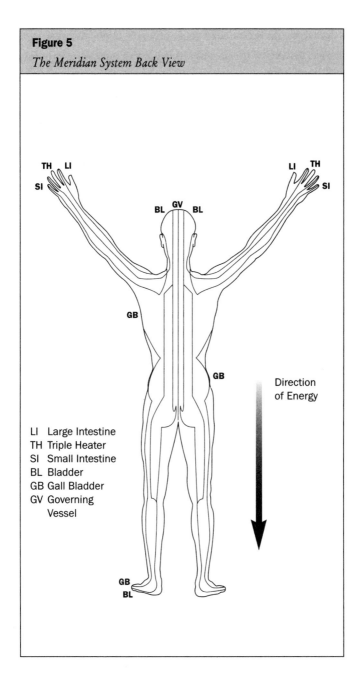

Figure 5

The Meridian System Back View

LI Large Intestine
TH Triple Heater
SI Small Intestine
BL Bladder
GB Gall Bladder
GV Governing
     Vessel

Direction
of Energy

negative mental states, and remove prevalent undesirable emotions and moods. One of the beautiful things about working with Energy is that it affects a person's physical, mental and spiritual state. As these different aspects of us are all composed of Energy, any change in Energy flow will have an effect at all levels of our being. Different people may be more aware of the benefits of a Shiatsu treatment at one or another level.

The different Energy systems in the human being are all inter-connected, so working on one Energy system will also affect all the others. So with Shiatsu working on the Meridian system, changes will also happen in the Chakras and subtle bodies.

Figure 6

The Cyclic Movement of Energy Through the Meridians

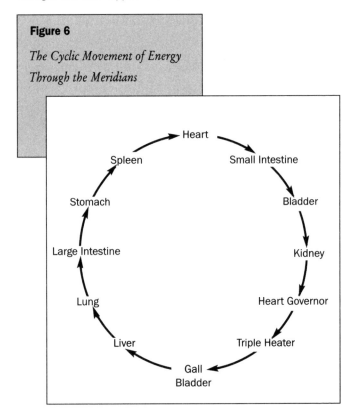

◆ Tsubos

The flow of Energy in the Meridians can be affected by giving pressure or other stimuli anywhere along the length of a Meridian travelling over the surface of the body. However, certain points on the Meridians have been found to be commonly most effective in changing the Energy flow in the Meridians, and so have the greatest beneficial effect in restoring health. These are the approximately 365 points used in acupuncture to insert needles.

In acupuncture and acupressure only these limited number of points are used. In Shiatsu the whole length of a Meridian is often worked on, and not just the acupuncture points. As well as using some of the acupuncture points, any point that feels imbalanced is held to affect the Energy at that point. In Shiatsu it is considered that there are an unlimited number of Tsubos, which can be found anywhere on the body.

Shiatsu uses a wide range of methods to beneficially affect the flow of Energy in the body, and is not restricted to just using the acupuncture points. However, some of the points are often included as part of a Shiatsu treatment. Chapter 11 will tell you how to find many of the commonly used points and the kinds of problems that they can be useful for. This chapter is placed towards the end of the book as you will find it much easier to find and use Tsubos after developing your sensitivity to Ki through practising full-body Shiatsu for a while.

◆ An Energetic Definition of Health

As we are working with Energy, we need to be able to define health in Energetic terms. An Energetic definition of physical, mental and spiritual health could be:

1. Having an approximately even distribution of Energy in all the

Meridians and other Energy systems; that is, the amount of Energy in all parts of the body is balanced.

Based on Figure 6 on page 30 showing the Energy flow through the twelve Meridians, this can be illustrated as:

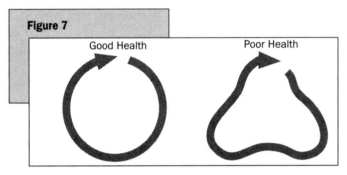

Figure 7

Good Health   Poor Health

When there is much more or less Energy in a Meridian or part of the body, physical and psychological symptoms arise. It never ceases to amaze me that when someone points out an area of pain, there is always an imbalance of Energy there (either too much or too little) and that simply redressing the balance causes the pain to disappear.

2. Energy is flowing, rather than being blocked or trapped. Life is Energy in movement. When Energy stops moving, then we become less alive, and our health is reduced. This can be illustrated as:

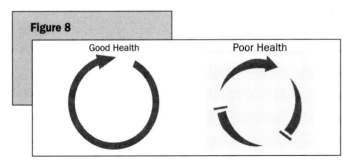

Figure 8

Good Health   Poor Health

3. Having a strong flow of Energy. The more Energy we have within us, the greater our physical vitality and stamina, mental positivity and clarity, and the wider and deeper our consciousness.

This definition of health may seem impossible to ever attain. This is true! We are used to a static definition of health, such as, 'the absence of any obvious symptoms or signs of illness'. With such a definition, either we are healthy or we are not. The above Energetic definition of health recognises that health is relative, that is, we can always improve our health. It is open-ended, and allows for us to continually increase our physical, mental and spiritual health.

◆ Working with Energy

From the Energetic definition of health, it is easy to see what we are trying to do in giving Shiatsu. We want to:

1. Rebalance the Energy in different Meridians and areas of the body – reducing the Energy where there is too much, and increasing the Energy where there is too little.

2. Where Energy has become stuck or blocked, get it moving.

3. Increase the total Energy within a person. One is quite limited in the amount one can do this in giving Shiatsu. The main ways of increasing our Energy are through our daily way of life, such as our choice of diet, full breathing, sufficient physical exercise, and a positive mental attitude. However, during the Shiatsu treatment described in this book a person becomes deeply relaxed, and in this state stops using up Energy and receives more from the outside. With regular Shiatsu a person can learn

to maintain a more relaxed state all the time. They will then not waste their Energy in unnecessary tension, and can continually receive more Energy from the outside.

When you begin giving Shiatsu, you may not be able to detect your friend's Energy clearly, so you will probably not feel where Energy is high or low or blocked. However, if you carefully follow the directions in this book, especially the Basic Principles, you will be working on a person's Energy, and you will automatically tend to rebalance their Energy and clear Energy blockages. Those receiving your Shiatsu will certainly feel the difference! With practise, areas of high and low Energy will begin to reveal themselves to you.

Chapter 3

EXERCISES TO PERCEIVE KI

H ere are a few exercises to enable you to feel Ki, so that it becomes more real for you. Most people who try these exercises for the first time can feel Ki. If you cannot, do not worry! It does not mean that you never will be able to, as everybody can learn to perceive Ki with a little practise. For all these exercises it helps if you are feeling calm and relaxed, and are in a quiet environment without distractions. For the second and third exercises you will need a partner.

◆ Exercise 1: Feeling Ki Between Your Hands

Stand with your feet about shoulder width apart and stretch your hands above your head. Now rub them together vigorously so that they become really warm and alive. Then also rub the backs of the hands and your wrists and forearms. Drop your hands to your sides, then shake them, throwing your hands away from you as if you were throwing water off your hands. Stretch your hands up above your head and repeat the rubbing, followed by the shaking. Now hold your hands out in front of you – they will feel warm and alive, due to the extra blood and Ki flow that you have generated in them.

Drop your hands to your sides, take a deep breath and relax your body as you breathe out. Repeat this two or three times. Hold your hands about three feet apart with the palms facing each other, relax, and let your mind become empty. Now focus your attention on the space between your hands, and slowly move the hands towards each other. Keep your awareness on any feelings between your hands. If your hands get very close, do not let them touch; take them back out to three feet apart and start again.

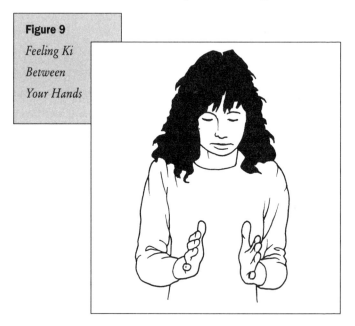

Figure 9

Feeling Ki Between Your Hands

When your hands get within six to twelve inches of each other you will probably feel some kind of sensation, such as warmth or tingling in your hands, or the feeling that you have an invisible bouncy balloon between your hands. This is the point at which the etheric aura of the two hands meet; the rubbing and shaking of the hands generated a stronger Energy field around your hands.

Take your hands out to three feet again and repeat the exercise until the feeling becomes more definite. When you get to the point of a definite feeling between your hands, play with it, moving your hands in and out slightly. Many people find their first sensation of Ki exciting!

◆ Exercise 2: Feeling Ki Around Another Person

Now we are going to repeat Exercise 1, but feeling the Ki around another person. Ask your partner to sit on a straight chair or on the floor. You are going to feel their etheric aura around their head and shoulders, as it is usually strongest and so easiest to feel here. Repeat the rubbing and shaking of your hands – the more Ki in your hands, the more sensitive you will be to perceiving Ki. Take a few deep breaths, and relax your body and mind as you breathe out. Now take one hand two or three feet to the side and above your partner's head, and slowly move your hand towards them. Focus your awareness on the space around their head. If you get very close to them, take your hand back out to two feet and start again.

Figure 10

Feeling Ki Around Another Person

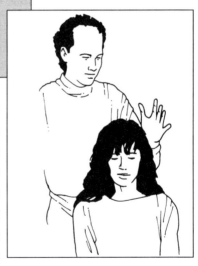

You will probably get a similar sensation as in Exercise 1 when you get two to six inches from the head. When you perceive their aura, move your hand in and out a little so as to repeatedly feel the boundary of the aura. Then you can work around the head and down over the shoulders, moving your hand out and in a little to keep feeling the aura. Keep going until the sensation becomes quite definite.

If you have difficulty feeling the aura, it is usually because the mind is too busy with thoughts. Relax yourself and let it settle down, then try the exercise again.

◆ Exercise 3: Directing Ki With The Mind

This exercise is a little different, but is interesting as it shows how we can control the Ki flow in our bodies to some extent with our minds. Get your partner to stand in front of you with their feet shoulder width apart. Put your arms around their hips and pick them up off the floor so that you can gauge their weight. Keep your back straight, and bend your knees to protect your own back. (Ideally choose a partner approximately the same weight as you. If you have back problems that may be aggravated by lifting, you had better not attempt this exercise.)

Now tell your partner to very slightly bend their knees (this automatically drops their Ki downwards into their abdomen) and to lean backwards a little so that they have more weight on their heels than on the balls of their feet (this encourages the flow of Ki down the back of the body. They should also look downwards towards the ground, and stay serious, as laughter or even a smile brings Energy upwards in the body. Then they can imagine themselves becoming very heavy, as heavy as lead. They can imagine Energy flowing down through their head, through their body, down their legs, and into the ground, making them heavier and rooted to the ground.

This visualization can be repeated for one or two minutes. Then, with your partner continuing their visualization, pick them up again. The difference in weight is generally obvious, often the partner is almost impossible to get off the ground!

Figure 11

Lifting a Partner

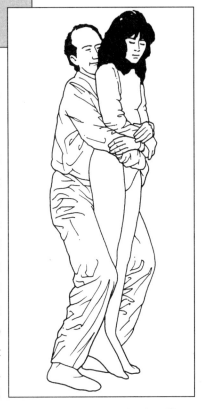

Now try the opposite, getting your partner to stand up straight, looking upwards with a smile, and with their weight tipped slightly forwards so that there is more weight on the balls of their feet than on their heels. They should imagine Energy flowing upwards from the ground into their feet, up through their legs, up the body, up through their head and out of the top of their head. This should be continued for one or two minutes, so that they feel as light as a feather. Then, with your partner continuing the visualization, slowly put your arms around their hips again and pick them up. Generally they will seem to fly into the air. Watch their head on the ceiling!

In this exercise you will feel how much your partner can change their weight by directing their Energy with their mind. The better their concentration, the bigger the difference you will feel in their weight when they make themselves heavy and light. You can swap around and try making yourself heavy and light for your partner to feel. Unfortunately for those who feel that they are overweight, visualizing being lighter does not alter the reading on weighing scales! A mechanical instrument does not register the difference in weight, only a human lifter who uses Ki to lift with. If you have spent time with children, you may have already noticed how a child that does not want to be picked up can make themselves feel very heavy. Some martial arts masters who are very practised in controlling their Ki can make themselves so heavy and rooted that even four people cannot pick them up.

Hopefully these three exercises have made the world of Ki more real to you. When giving Shiatsu, variations in the amount of Energy in different areas of the body and in different Meridians and Tsubos can be clearly felt. Unfortunately this can be difficult at first because one is touching the receiver's body, and the physical sensation of touching tends to dominate the sensing of Ki. With practise in giving Shiatsu everyone can learn to feel Ki too.

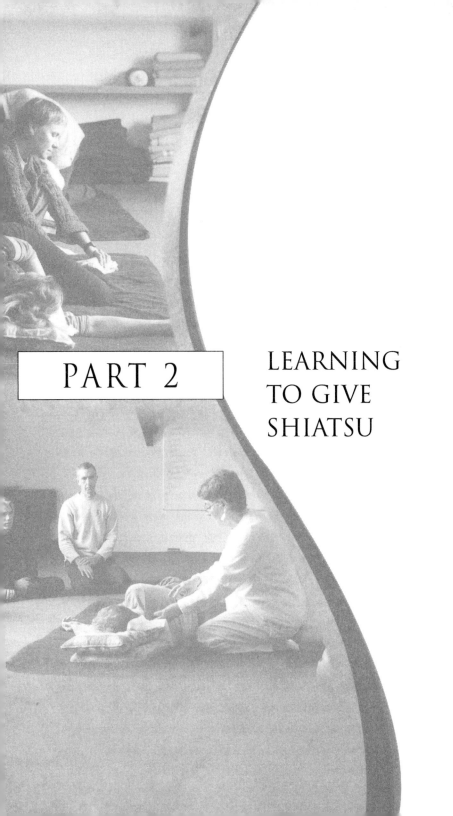

PART 2

LEARNING TO GIVE SHIATSU

Chapter 4

PRACTICAL DETAILS

◆ Preparations for Giving Shiatsu

Shiatsu has the great advantage of needing no equipment – just your hands which you carry everywhere with you! So you can give Shiatsu almost anywhere, at any time. However, the following guidelines for ideal preparations and environment will enable you to give better Shiatsu and for the receiver to benefit more from treatment.

1. The ideal clothing for both the giver and receiver is a single layer of loose cotton clothing, such as a track or jogging suit, or a T-shirt and loose pair of thin cotton trousers (not jeans!). Ki does not flow easily through artificial fibred clothing, so if they are worn by the receiver, it will be more difficult for you to make contact with their Ki. If you wear artificial fibres, your Ki cannot flow so easily, making your Shiatsu less effective. It is also advisable to wear natural fibres – cotton, wool, silk or flax – for normal daily wear to allow your Energy to move more freely around the body and between your body and the environment. Remember, life is Energy, so if you constrict or cut down on the Energy you receive, you will feel less alive. This is more important for clothing worn directly against the skin, such as underwear, stockings, trousers or shirts. For Shiatsu the clothing must also be loose to allow you to move freely when giving Shiatsu, and for you to be able to move the receiver's body freely when giving stretches.

2. The room you are giving Shiatsu in should be quite warm, as the receiver usually cools down a lot as they relax. If it is warm enough, you will probably want to be wearing only light clothing yourself. If you think the room may be a little cool, have a blanket handy, and while you are giving Shiatsu to the upper body you can cover the lower body, and when you move onto the lower body, cover the upper body.

3. Unlike some forms of massage, Shiatsu is ideally given with the receiver lying on a mat on the floor. This allows the giver to use their weight effortlessly to give Shiatsu, rather than their muscular strength. The mat needs to be soft enough to make the receiver comfortable, but also firm so that the weight given on the body does not get taken up by the mat instead of affecting the receiver. Two to four blankets, folded in half if necessary, with a clean sheet over them is good to begin with. A Japanese futon (a thin all-cotton mattress) one to three layers thick is ideal.

4. The room must give enough space for the receiver to lie down, and for you to be able to move freely all around them. This means three or four feet at their head and feet and to their sides.

5. The room should be clean and tidy. Looking at this Energetically, dust and dirt are stores of stagnant Ki that will subtly block the Ki flow of the giver and receiver. If belongings are chaotically or messily left around the room, their chaotic Ki will subtly interfere with your concentration and focus during the Shiatsu. A clean, orderly room allows your Ki to move clearly. This of course applies to your daily living space as much as it does to the place you prepare for giving Shiatsu.

6. Have one or two cushions handy in case your friend is uncomfortable lying on the mat. For example, lying face down with the head turned to the left or right can cause some people's necks to become stiff or painful. Often they do not realize until they come to turn over onto their back, when there is a shriek of pain! To prevent this put a cushion under one shoulder, and tell them to turn their head towards the cushion. The cushion could also be put under the upper chest.

   If people have stiffness in the knees, cushions can be placed under the lower legs. Sometimes when people lie on their back a small cushion is needed under the lower back to prevent pain.

7. The room should be as quiet as possible. Noise tends to distract you, and can prevent the receiver fully relaxing. You may need to take the telephone off the hook, and to put a 'do not disturb' notice up on the door. Some people like to play some quiet, relaxing music while giving Shiatsu.

8. Make sure your fingernails are cut short. You do not want to give acupuncture instead of Shiatsu! Long nails can be quite painful for the receiver.

9. Do anything else you think of to increase the comfort and relaxation of the receiver, and your easy movement and concentration.

◆ When Not To Give Shiatsu

There are some situations when it is advisable not to give Shiatsu.

1. If you or the receiver have had a large, heavy meal, wait several hours before giving Shiatsu. The Ki in you or your

friend's body will be directed inwards for the digestion of the food, so less Ki will be circulating around the body in the Meridians, making the giving or receiving of Shiatsu less effective. It is fine to give or receive Shiatsu after eating lightly.

2. Don't give pressure on recently broken bones, varicose veins, deep cuts, or other injuries. The receiver probably won't appreciate your resetting their fracture!

3. Shiatsu can be very helpful during pregnancy, especially for relieving the back pains that often arise. However there are certain areas on the body that give strong stimulation to the womb. Shiatsu on these places can be useful during labour to stimulate stronger contractions, but should not be used during pregnancy. These areas are:
   a) The ankles. In fact it is safest not to give any heavy pressure to the feet or legs below the knees.
   b) The fleshy area on the hands between the thumb and the base of the first finger.
   c) The top of the shoulders just either side of the neck.
   d) The abdomen.

4. If someone has been rushing about, or is feeling very emotional, give them a little time to calm down before giving them Shiatsu. Directing them to take some long, deep breaths will help them to calm down more quickly.

   In addition, people with certain problems or conditions may be helped by an experienced Shiatsu practitioner, but should not be given Shiatsu by someone just beginning to learn Shiatsu.

5. Do not give Shiatsu for at least several weeks after a person has had an operation, or after a woman has given birth.

6. Avoid giving Shiatsu to people with serious health problems such as cancer, multiple sclerosis, severe arthritis, heart problems, etc. Shiatsu can be very helpful for these people, but a precise diagnosis and treatment is needed. People with serious health problems are often very low in overall Ki, with big imbalances between different areas and Meridians. An inaccurate Shiatsu could deplete them of Energy, or worsen symptoms. You could try just doing their hands and feet.

    There may also be people who do not have any obvious symptoms or named illness, but who appear to you to be ill looking. These people may well be building up big health problems, which haven't yet surfaced to create definite symptoms. If you feel uneasy about giving such a person Shiatsu, follow your intuition and don't give them Shiatsu.

Remember, before you give anyone Shiatsu, ask them if they have any health problems, and if they are pregnant. And if you are in any doubt about whether or not you should give them Shiatsu, don't.

◆ Possible Effects of Your Shiatsu Treatment

Most people will feel relaxed and rejuvenated after your Shiatsu. Beneficial effects of the Shiatsu may be noticed days or even weeks later, so make a point of always asking people a few days after the Shiatsu if they have noticed any changes. This is very useful feedback for you. Commonly reported changes include feeling more relaxed, sleeping better, being more flexible with the release of areas of tension, feeling lighter and more alive, or that a weight has been lifted from them, and the disappearance of minor problems like backache or tired eyes.

A few people may experience changes that do not seem so welcome. It will help you to know of the most common reactions, and their probable causes.

1. *Tiredness.* Many people will take five or ten minutes to come out of their deep relaxation, and to be ready to take on the world again. This is natural. A few people feel exhausted, and want to do nothing but have a long sleep. These are generally people who keep going on 'nervous tension', which is actually tension in the body. When Shiatsu removes the tension, a state of underlying tiredness or need to rest is revealed. You can advise these people to rest or sleep until they feel recuperated. Unfortunately this is not always possible with the hectic pace of modern life.

2. *Coughing, mucus or colds.* During or after the Shiatsu a person may begin coughing, or producing mucus from the nose. Rarely this may turn into a cold. What is happening here is that the body has been stimulated to discharge some of the excess fats, sugars, and other foods eaten in the form of mucus. As practically everyone in modern society has a good deal of excess in their bodies, the discharge of some of this excess is a welcome event.

    Sometimes, when mucus is present, a cold virus is able to infect the body, giving symptoms like aching, tiredness and coldness. It should be realized, though, that the cold virus is not so much the cause of the problem, as the result. Only when body cells are in a less healthy state will they be susceptible to infection by the cold virus or any other virus. So if somebody starts discharging mucus or develops a cold after receiving Shiatsu, you can explain that this is beneficial for their health!

3. *Headaches, other aches and pains.* Occasionally a person will develop a headache or aches or pains in other parts of their body after Shiatsu. Generally they last no longer than twenty-four hours. There are two common causes of this. Firstly, Shiatsu can release Ki that has been locked up in areas of tension for a long time. When this Ki is released, it can surge around the body until it settles down to a new balance. While the Ki is surging, an excess or deficiency of Ki may temporarily occur in a part of the body, causing an ache or pain. You can reassure the person that the pain is part of a process of the body moving to a state of greater balance and health.

   A second common cause of pain is that you have worked too hard or too long on a particular part of the body. The ideal amount of pressure to give to the body varies widely between different people. You can imagine that a small, frail elderly person would need a lot less pressure than a large, muscular young adult. In the exercises of the next chapter you will learn how to gauge how much pressure to give, so that this is unlikely to happen.

   A particular case is someone who regularly has headaches or migraines. It can be tempting to spend longer or to give more pressure on the head in an effort to help them. However this can bring on a headache, by bringing more Ki to the head where there is already an excess. It is more important to relax the shoulders and neck, and give Shiatsu to the whole body. Even without touching the head these people can be helped by full-body Shiatsu rebalancing Ki in the whole body.

If a headache or pain persists for longer than two or three days, it would be advisable for the person to seek guidance from a qualified Shiatsu practitioner or other health professional.

4. *Release of emotions.* Every area of tension or weakness in the body is associated with certain held emotions, feelings and thoughts. When a person's Ki is stimulated to move and rebalance, they may experience these emotions. Often they may relate to some event in the past when the person experienced a strong emotion, but instead of expressing it or resolving it inwardly, they suppressed it. During the Shiatsu it is generally beneficial for people to express any strong feelings or emotions that come up, so that they can be got rid of for good. A little gentle encouragement from you can be a lot of help to them in this. Some people may want a good cry, and can be given some warm comfort.

5. *Feeling nothing at all.* Occasionally, when asked, a person will say that they haven't felt any effects at all from your Shiatsu. This can be very discouraging when you are just beginning to learn Shiatsu. However, don't be put off! This comment usually says more about the person than about your Shiatsu. Many people are quite 'disconnected' from their bodies, with little awareness of areas of tension, weakness or other sensation. Only when they experience strong pain do they realize that something is wrong. So they will be unlikely to consciously register the effects of your Shiatsu, even though it may have been beneficial. Shiatsu can be a useful way of helping these people to get more in touch with their bodies. Encourage them to be more aware of your touch and the effects it has.

One cause of this insensitivity is eating a typical modern

diet, high in animal fats. As the body cannot use up all of the fat, it accumulates in and around the organs of the body, and also under the skin. These fat deposits act as a great insulator to Ki, blocking its flow. Shiatsu is generally less effective for people with much fat accumulation, as it is that much more difficult to get the body's Ki flowing. You may have to work with as much weight as you can, still to be told by the receiver that they can't feel anything! The Shiatsu technique of walking on the receiver's back was probably invented for these kinds of people!

If someone experiences these, or other seemingly unwelcome effects from your Shiatsu, explain to them the probable causes of their symptoms. This can make them feel a lot happier about Shiatsu, rather then being left with a bad impression.

Chapter 5

PRELIMINARY EXERCISES

In learning the practical side of giving Shiatsu, this is a very important chapter. By practising these exercises you will learn how to use your Ki to affect a receiver's Ki. In the next chapter we will look at the techniques used in giving Shiatsu. For these outward techniques to be effective, it is important that you are using your Ki, and not just performing them physically.

During these exercises you will be introduced to some Basic Principles for Giving Shiatsu. When you are following these Basic Principles you will be primarily using your Ki to give Shiatsu, rather than your physical power, and you will automatically primarily affect the receiver's Ki, rather than their physical body. So even though you may not yet be sensitive to your friend's Ki, you will be moving and balancing their Ki. Good reports from those receiving your Shiatsu will be evidence of this.

◆ Exercise 1: Abdominal Breathing

We have three main centres in the body, as shown in Figure 12. The **ABDOMINAL CENTRE** relates to the lower three Chakras and is concerned with our individual existence on Earth. When there is a lot of Energy in the abdominal centre we feel centred and grounded, confident, calm and peaceful, with plenty of physical vitality.

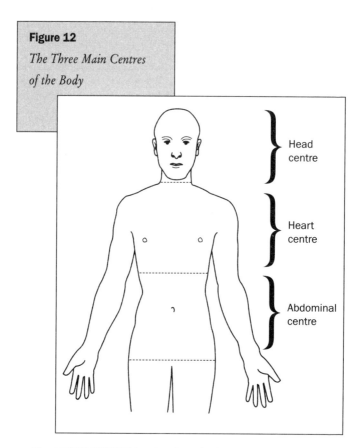

Figure 12

The Three Main Centres of the Body

Head centre

Heart centre

Abdominal centre

The **HEART CENTRE** is related to the heart and throat Chakras, and is concerned with our relations to other people, to nature, and the outside world. When this area is active we feel more love, empathy and compassion for people.

The **HEAD CENTRE** relates to the brow Chakra and to mental activity. This may be more intellectual, analytical thinking or more imaginative and intuitive thinking.

When we are physically active our Energy moves into the abdominal centre. When we are interacting with other people in an open-hearted way, Energy moves more to the heart centre. When we are thinking a lot, Energy gathers in our head. (Thinking too much or for too long can create a headache caused by an excess of Energy in the head.)

Ideally our Energy should be approximately evenly distributed between these three centres, giving a balanced life with the practical, social and mental aspects of life all fulfilled. However this is often not the case. Due to differences in diet, activity, education, social norms, and other factors, particular centres may be over or underactive. Some people are 'all in their heads', others are 'all heart', and some are 'doers' without much thought or heart.

Different cultures often have broadly different Energy distributions (this partly accounts for the difficulty that is often experienced in communication between different cultures). Modern Western culture puts a lot of emphasis on mental development, whereas Far Eastern cultures traditionally put greater emphasis on developing centredness and groundedness. People from tropical and sub-tropical countries are often much more emotional and open about their feelings than people living in colder climates.

Shiatsu, coming from Japan, puts greater emphasis on centering in the abdominal centre. In Japanese the abdomen is called the *Hara*. This is a very useful practice for us generally head centred Westerners, and is one of the great benefits of learning Shiatsu. Here we are going to use our breath to change our Energy distribution in our body. When we breathe in, we not only take in oxygen, but also Ki, from the air. The air and oxygen is taken into our lungs, but with our minds we can direct the Ki to any part of the body we choose, to strengthen the Ki in that area. With abdominal breathing we direct this Ki to the Hara, to increase our centredness, groundedness and vitality.

Abdominal breathing is ideally practised just before giving a Shiatsu treatment. However, if you practise it for five minutes a day, say after getting up in the morning, for a period of one to two months, your Energy can permanently become more centred in the Hara. This will make you feel more grounded with more vitality during your normal daily activities, which can make a real difference to your experience of daily life. And once you have got the hang of the exercise, you can practise it at almost any time, standing in a bus queue, sitting at work, while washing up, or when driving a car. Any time you feel flustered, tired, or uptight, it can help you become calm and centred in dealing with the daily challenges of life.

The Exercise

For this exercise you need to sit with a straight back, to maximize the Ki taken into the Spiritual Channel. If you can, sit in *seiza*, as shown in the illustration, the traditional Japanese way of sitting.

However if this position is uncomfortable, sit cross-legged with a cushion under your bottom, or on a staight-backed chair. Put your hands together in your lap. Take a few deep breaths and relax your body and mind as you breathe out. We will now build up to the full exercise in stages.

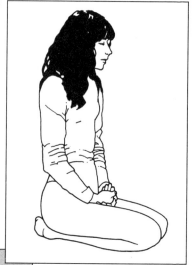

Figure 13 *Sitting in Seiza*

Stage 1

Place one hand on your chest and the other on your abdomen below the navel. You are now going to breathe with just your abdomen, and not with the chest. Take a slow breath in, keeping your chest still, and allowing your abdomen to expand. Then relax, letting the air out, with your abdomen falling inwards. Repeat this breathing for two or three minutes, then take a rest and practise it again. Breathe as deeply as you can while keeping the chest still, by expanding the abdomen as much as possible – it feels a bit like blowing a balloon up as far as possible.

Some people find breathing using only their abdomen quite easy straight away, for others it can be a difficult exercise. One reason for this is that in modern culture we are unconsciously taught to breathe more superficially only into the chest. (This makes our perceptions, thinking and living more superficial, compared with also using our abdomen which makes us more rooted, with deeper and wider perceptions and thinking. If you watch babies breathing, they mostly use their abdomens.) Another reason for difficulty in practising abdominal breathing is tension in the diaphragm, the sheet of muscle at the bottom of the rib cage separating the lungs from the abdominal organs, or general stiffness in the liver, stomach, intestines, and other organs in the abdomen.

Practise stage 1 until it is easy for you, and you can do it with your hands in your lap instead of on your chest and abdomen. Then progress to stage 2.

Stage 2

Place the palm of one hand over the area below your navel, and the other hand on top of the first hand. Take a slow breath in through the nose, and visualise the air travelling down through your body to the Hara beneath your hands. You may like to close your eyes to aid concentration on the visualization.

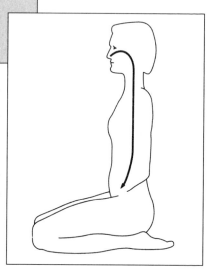

Figure 14

Breathing Ki into the Hara

Hold your breath for three or four seconds, keeping your attention on the Ki gathered in your Hara. Then slowly let the air trickle out of your mouth (you lose less of the Ki breathing out of the mouth in this way than if you breathed out of the nose). Repeat this breathing for two or three minutes, visualizing the Ki travelling down to your Hara with each in breath.

Slowly open your eyes, look around, and observe how you feel. Different? Practise abdominal breathing regularly, and these effects will become a more permanent part of your being.

◆ Exercise 2: Centred Movement on the Floor

Abdominal breathing helps to centre our Ki in the Hara. Now we are going to practise moving from this centre, so that we use our Ki to give Shiatsu rather than our physical, muscular strength. When we use our Ki to give Shiatsu, we primarily affect the Ki of the receiver. Also, after giving Shiatsu, rather than feeling tired from exertion, one feels uplifted and energized from the increased Ki flow in oneself. This is one of the great rewards in giving Shiatsu. We get as much from giving a Shiatsu as the receiver!

The Exercise

'Stand' on your all-fours, that is on your hands and knees. Have your hands and knees about shoulder width apart, with your arms either straight or almost straight, whichever is most comfortable. Relax! Let your body flop as much as possible while holding this position. Check that you are not tensing your shoulders, back, neck or arms. You are now giving perfect Shiatsu to the floor!

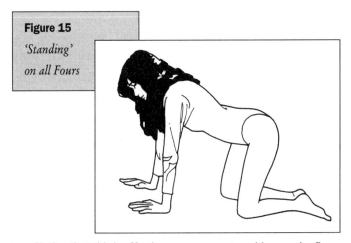

Figure 15
'Standing' on all Fours

Notice that this is effortless – you are not pushing on the floor, just resting your weight on it. And there is no need for any tension in your body. You are now experiencing the first three Basic Principles of giving Shiatsu:

1. **Use your weight, and not your strength.**

2. **Give Shiatsu effortlessly.**

3. **Stay relaxed, don't tense up.**

This may seem strange to you, as we are so used to making effort to achieve various aims or goals in our lives. What you are learning through this exercise, and will learn further through giving Shiatsu, is that life need not be a constant struggle, requiring endless effort and strain. The whole of life can become an easy flow from one activity to the next.

Now let's practise moving. Rock your weight forwards a little so that you are putting more weight on the floor through your hands. Now slowly rock your weight more onto your left hand, then your left hand and knee, then both knees, then your right knee, and onto your right knee and hand, then onto the right hand, and finally back to both hands.

To make these movements you will have been moving your whole body, with the movement centred on your Hara. Make another half dozen or so slow circles, then do about the same number in the opposite direction, moving clockwise rather than anti-clockwise. Then come back to the central all-fours position.

While you are moving, observe yourself following the first three Basic Principles, using your weight effortlessly and without tension. Furthermore, notice that to change the weight you are giving to the floor through your hands, you move your whole body, and that your body's centre of gravity is in the abdomen. You are experiencing the fourth Basic Principle:

4. Change your weight on the receiver by moving your whole body, with your Hara as the centre of movement.

Now rock your body forwards to increase the weight your hands are giving to the floor, hold the position for four or five seconds, then rock backwards with more weight on your knees. Rock forwards onto your hands again, hold for four or five seconds, then rock back. Repeat this about a dozen times, observing how with your whole body movement you increase and decrease the weight you are giving to the floor through your hands. Then come back to the central position. You have now been following two more of the Basic Principles:

5. **Use your weight at right-angles to the body surface. (In this exercise, the floor.)**

6. **Hold your weight on the receiver for a short time.**

The reason for always using your weight at right-angles to the body surface is that you then contact the body's Ki. Coming in at an angle you will have much less effect on a person's Ki flow. As the body is rounded, unlike the floor, you will need to adjust your position so that you are always effortlessly using your weight at right-angles to the receiver's body surface.

When you are leaning your weight on a person or giving a stretch, the position is held for a short time, usually between five and fifteen seconds. This is because the movement of increasing your weight on a person has a more physical effect, but while you hold still, Ki moves within the receiver. So, if we want to work with Energy, we hold in most techniques. While holding a position, there is a particular moment when the place you are holding or stretching 'opens', and a lot of Energy moves at once. The time taken for this opening to happen usually lies between three and twenty seconds. If you don't hold, this opening and movement of Energy never happens.

It is unlikely that you will feel this opening phenomenon when you first practise Shiatsu, so I advise that you generally hold all movements for four or five seconds.

◆ Exercise 3: Centred Movement on a Partner

Now we are going to practise applying the Basic Principles giving
Shiatsu to another person instead of the floor! Ask your partner to
lie down on their front on a mat or several blankets. Move their left
arm away from their body so it lies approximately at right-angles
to their body, then kneel on their left side facing at right-angles to
the line of their body. Take up the all-fours position as before, with
your right hand on the hard sacrum between their hips, and your
left hand between their shoulder blades. You should feel exactly
the same as when you were on all-fours on the floor – relaxed, with
arms straight or just slightly bent, resting your weight on them
effortlessly. (It is amazing how at this point the mind can start
thinking, 'I must do something now', and one starts tensing up and
using muscular effort!)

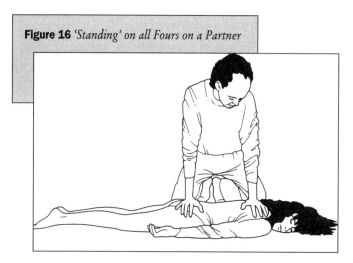

Figure 16 *'Standing' on all Fours on a Partner*

Rock your weight back a little onto your knees, then forwards
onto your hands, and hold for four or five seconds. Then rock back
onto your knees, then forwards again and hold. Repeat this simple
movement about a dozen times, checking that you are:

1. Using your weight and not your strength.
2. Moving effortlessly.
3. Staying relaxed.
4. Moving your whole body.
5. Giving your weight at right-angles to their back.
6. Holding your weight for four or five seconds each time you lean forwards.

Also, ask your partner if you are using too little or too much weight. If you are using too little the Shiatsu can feel ineffective. To increase the weight on your hands, move your body further forwards over their body to increase the weight on your hands. If your partner is large, muscular, or in good health, you may need to move your knees back further away from them so that you can give more weight through your hands.

If you are using too much weight, your partner will say it hurts! Generally one does not want to cause pain when giving Shiatsu, as it makes the receiver tense up, and this tension prevents their Ki flowing. So ease up and use a little less weight, that is don't move your body so far forwards onto your hands.

When students first practise this exercise, they often give too little weight. It can be quite surprising just how much weight you can use when you are in this relaxed state. So keep asking your partner for feedback, and experiment with using different amounts of weight to find the middle point between being ineffectual and causing pain or discomfort. At this middle point you will be giving Shiatsu most effectively.

This middle point will obviously vary a lot with different people. Generally larger, more muscular, fitter, and younger adults need more weight, and with smaller, frailer, less fit, and older adults or children less weight is needed. However, the best thing to do at first is to ask the people you are giving Shiatsu to what feels right for them. This is more accurate than guessing!

When you find the middle point in this exercise, you can then lean your weight onto your partner confidently. This is very important, because if you are hesitating or holding back for fear of hurting them, you will also be withholding your Ki. This makes the Shiatsu less effective. This is just the same as any action in life – if we do something 'wholeheartedly' and with 'body and soul', we not only enjoy ourselves more, but also achieve far more. So find the right weight for your partner, and then lean your weight on them with body, heart and soul!

The middle point or right amount of weight will obviously be different for each part of the body. Large structures like the back, thighs and bottom usually need a lot of weight, and smaller and softer structures like the ankles, hands, abdomen and face need less. So the first few times you practise the full-body Shiatsu treatment described in the next chapter, you will probably need to keep asking your partner if you are using too little or too much weight. This may seem to break into the flow of the Shiatsu, but is well worth doing at first so that you quickly learn to make your Shiatsu as effective as possible. With time you will develop the sensitivity to know how much weight to use for a particular person and part of the body through the feel of the place you are working.

That's enough on weight! Now rock forwards and backwards a few more times, ensuring that you are giving equal weight on both hands. Don't be biased towards either hand. You are now experiencing another Basic Principle, that when using two hands to give Shiatsu:

7. Use equal weight on both hands.

Having practised your own movement, we are now going to progress to moving your hands over the receiver. The right hand will stay in the same place on the sacrum while the left hand moves down the back, giving Shiatsu to the large muscles lying either side of the spine. Put the heel of your left hand about 1¹/₂ inches to the right of the spine, between the shoulder blades. Let the palm and fingers rest on the back. Now rock your body forwards, giving equal weight through your right hand and heel of your left hand, hold for four or five seconds, then rock backwards.

Figure 17 *Palming Down the Back*

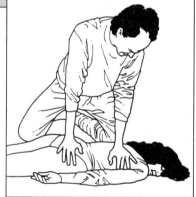

Move your left hand down the back about a hand's width, rock forwards and hold, then rock back. Move your left hand down another hand's width, and continue down the back until your left hand reaches the hip.

Take your left hand back up to the level of the shoulder blades and repeat the Shiatsu down the right side of the receiver's back. If you are unsure about how much weight to use, ask your partner how it feels.

Having worked down the right side twice, place the heel of your left hand about 1¹/₂ inches to the left of the spine between the shoulder blades. Give Shiatsu to the left side of the spine twice, as you did for the right side.

Your partner should now be feeling wonderful! From practising this first Shiatsu form, you can appreciate another Basic Principle:

8. Move with a steady rhythm throughout your Shiatsu treatment. Besides the specific effects of the various forms used in a Shiatsu treatment, the rhythm of your movement throughout the Shiatsu has a big effect. If you slow up and spend too long working on one area, your Ki flow and the Ki flow of the receiver tends to slow up, and you will not be so effective in getting their Energy moving. If you go too quickly the receiver will probably not relax, and without proper holding the Shiatsu will only have a superficial effect. Between these two extremes is a comfortable, natural rhythm and effortless flow, rather like the feeling of rocking a baby. This will make the receiver feel very nurtured and open to your loving touch!

There is one more Basic Principle, which applies to the overall Shiatsu treatment:

9. Keep in contact with the receiver throughout the Shiatsu. When you are moving your own body around the receiver to give Shiatsu to different areas you may take both hands off them for several seconds. Try to avoid this. While you are moving yourself, keep one hand lightly on them. You may need to slide a hand from one area to the next to keep in contact. When a person becomes deeply relaxed during a Shiatsu session, prolonged loss of contact can give a slightly unpleasant feeling of being deserted. You do not have to be religious about this – a second's loss of contact will not matter, but five or ten seconds will.

If you have incorporated the Basic Principles into your Shiatsu, you will already be giving fine Shiatsu. If you are still a little unsure about using them, go through the exercises in this chapter again. Here are the Basic Principles again for you to refer to:

◆ The Basic Principles for Giving Shiatsu

1. Use your weight, and not your strength.

2. Give Shiatsu effortlessly.

3. Stay relaxed, don't tense up.

4. Change your weight on the receiver by moving your whole body, with your Hara as the centre of the movement.

5. Use your weight at right-angles to the body surface.

6. Hold your weight for a short time.

7. Use equal weight on both hands.

8. Move with a steady rhythm throughout your Shiatsu.

9. Keep in contact with the receiver throughout your Shiatsu.

Chapter 6

A BASIC SHIATSU SEQUENCE

Now that you have practised how to give Shiatsu, we can look at some techniques used in giving Shiatsu. In this chapter a number of basic techniques are described to make up a full-body Shiatsu treatment. There are hundreds of different techniques used in Shiatsu. Those presented here are a selection of those most commonly used. Once you have become proficient in using these, you can learn more from other books or by attending courses in Shiatsu.

Before you begin giving Shiatsu, remember the following points.

1. Don't forget to ask the receiver if they have any health problems to check if it is OK for you to give them Shiatsu, as described in Chapter 4.

2. Try to follow the directions on different techniques exactly. In each technique you should feel comfortable and relaxed. If the position feels awkward or difficult to maintain, try shifting your position around until you feel comfortable. Only when you are relaxed will your Ki flow and will your Shiatsu be effective.

3. When you are leaning your weight on the receiver or giving a stretch, hold the position for three to five seconds. As you practise this full-body Shiatsu treatment, you may sometimes feel that

you want to hold for a longer time in certain areas. Follow this intuition, and hold for as long as you feel appropriate.

4. Each technique can be performed once, or several times. To begin with, do each technique once unless the directions state otherwise. Again as you practise giving this full-body treatment you may sometimes feel like repeating a technique two or three times – follow your intuition.

5. When you are giving pressure on the receiver's back, abdomen or chest, you should increase the pressure while they breathe out, and then reduce the pressure long enough for him or her to breathe in. If you can't see his or her breathing, then tell them when to breathe in and out. It helps if you breathe with them. You will probably find that you naturally begin to breathe out whenever you lean your weight or move into a technique, synchronizing your breathing with all your movements.

6. It is difficult to describe how much weight your should use when giving Shiatsu. Generally, if you are relaxed and not using force, you will probably be able to use more weight than you might think. With practise you will develop 'the feel' for what is the right pressure for a certain place on the body of a particular person. However at first it can be difficult to judge, so ask the receiver for feedback 'is this too hard?', 'am I using enough weight?', or simply, 'how does this feel?'.

7. With a little practise this full-body treatment should last about forty to fifty minutes. It may take you a little longer at first. However, if you continue to take over an hour to complete it, you are probably going too slowly, and not keeping up a good pace or rhythm through your Shiatsu.

◆ The Back and Shoulders

1. Begin by kneeling on the left side of the receiver. Put your right hand on his or her sacrum, and pause for a few seconds while you become calm and centred. 'Tune in' to the person's body, emotions and thoughts.

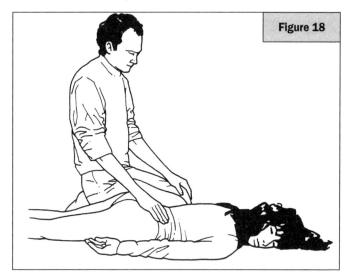

Figure 18

2. Keeping your hand on the sacrum, palm down the far side of the back twice, and then down the near side twice. Begin between the shoulder blades and continue down to the small of the back.

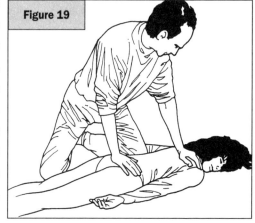

Figure 19

3. Step across the receiver, and position their arms with the palm upwards and the elbows slightly bent. Put the palm of your left hand between the spine and shoulder blade, and with the other hand palm twice down the whole length of the arm and onto the palm of the hand. You may well feel tension in the shoulder relax as you work down the arm. Now repeat this on the other arm.

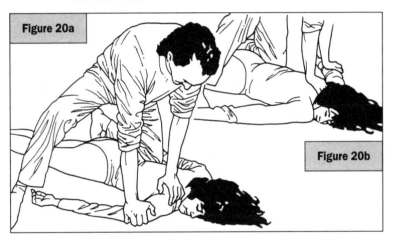

Figure 20a

Figure 20b

4. Place your thumbs close to the spine between the shoulders.

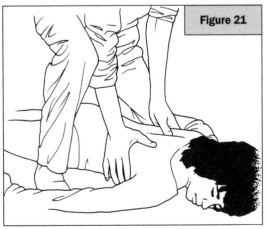

Figure 21

Steady your thumbs by giving firm pressure with your fingers also. Lean your weight forwards and hold for a few seconds. Move your thumbs down an inch and repeat. Continue down the back, and then on to the bony sacrum.

5. Bring one arm up over the back, and hold in place at the elbow with your knee or foot. Pull the shoulder up as you lean your weight downwards through your fingers, pressing under the shoulder blade. Repeat several times, working your fingers under the bottom and top of the shoulder blade.

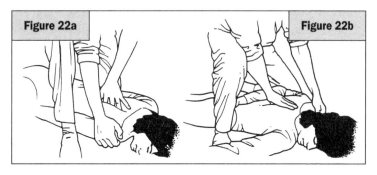

Figure 22a   Figure 22b

6. Release the arm, hold onto the wrist and raise the arm. Turn the arm so that the little finger points towards their head – this locks the elbow. Hold the shoulder firmly with the other hand and rotate the arm in little circles to loosen the shoulder. Then move the arm towards the receiver's head until you feel some resistance, and hold this stretch for a few seconds. *Be Gentle!* It is easy to go too far and cause pain. Rotate the arm a few times and repeat the stretch. Place the arm on the floor and repeat stages 5 and 6 on the other arm.

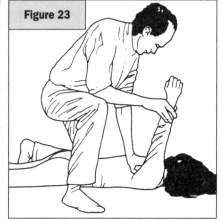

Figure 23

◆ The Buttocks

7. Move down to the receiver's hips, and with one hand on the sacrum, palm one buttock. Start at the top of the buttock and work down to the top of the leg.

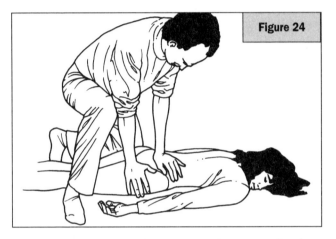

Figure 24

8. Keep the same hand on the sacrum, and use your thumb to press three or four points down a line through the centre of the buttock.

9. Put your other hand on the sacrum and repeat stages 7 and 8 on the other buttock.

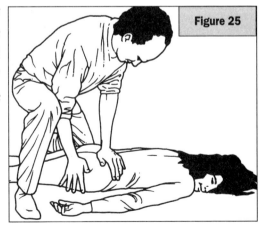

Figure 25

◆ The Legs

10. Bring your leg back so that you are kneeling beside the receiver. With your left hand on the sacrum, palm down one leg from the top to the ankle, moving your hand down about a palm's width each time. Quite a lot of weight can be given on the legs, but only light pressure can be used on and just above and below the knee otherwise you will hurt the front of the knee. If the receiver has long legs or if you have short arms, you may need to move the hand on the sacrum down to the upper leg.

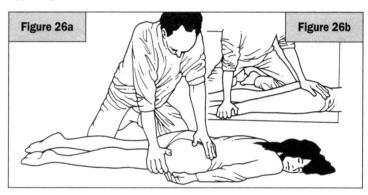

Figure 26a

Figure 26b

11. Put your moving hand on the heel, and lean forwards to stretch the inside of the lower leg.

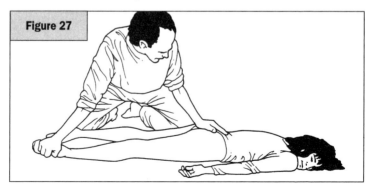

Figure 27

12. Repeat stages 10 and 11 on the other leg.

13. Move to between the receiver's legs, and with one hand on the sacrum, raise the lower leg holding onto the foot. Lean your weight onto both hands, giving a good stetch to the front of the thigh and lower leg. Remember to hold for a few seconds. If the foot easily reaches the bottom the receiver won't be getting much of a stretch, so move the foot to the outside of the bottom.

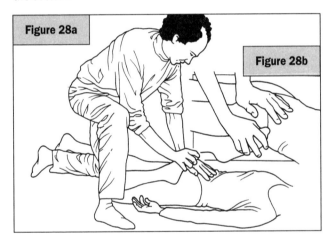

Figure 28a

Figure 28b

14. Bring the leg back so that the lower leg is vertical. Place one hand on the ball of the foot, and lean most of your weight onto it to stretchthe Achilles tendon. Place the foot back on the floor.

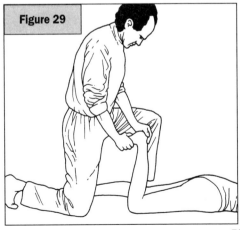

Figure 29

15. Repeat stages 13 and 14 on the other leg. You should hardly have to shift your own position while doing these stretches on the legs.

◆ Turning Over

Now ask your friend to turn over, slowly. He or she will probably be quite relaxed by now, so you don't want them to suddenly jump up and disturb this relaxation.

◆ The Feet

16. Kneel at the feet and, taking one foot, hold onto the back of the heel and press your thumb along three lines on the sole of the foot, holding each position for a few seconds.

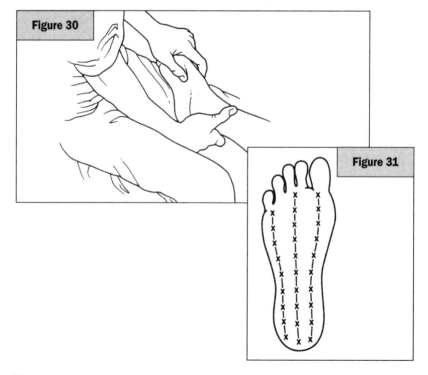

Figure 30

Figure 31

17. Stretch open the top of the foot by pressing down with the heels of your hands and pressing up with your fingers. This releases tension held in the top of the foot.

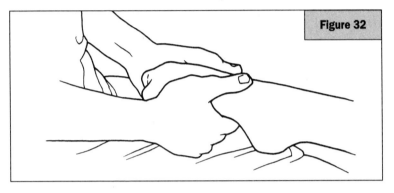

Figure 32

18. Stretch the toes upwards, and then downwards (carefully, as some people's toes don't stretch downwards very far). Repeat a few times to stretch the top and bottom of the foot.

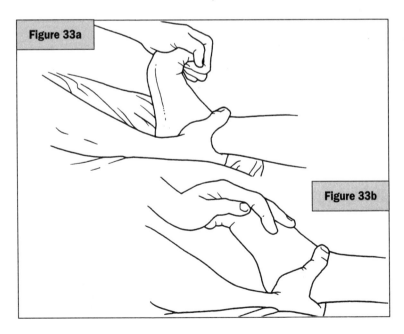

Figure 33a

Figure 33b

19. Hold onto the foot firmly with one hand, and hold the base of the little toe firmly between your thumb and first finger. Rotate the toe to loosen its joint with the foot, then lean back and stretch the toe away from the leg. You may get a crack as stagnant Energy is released. Do the same for all the other toes.

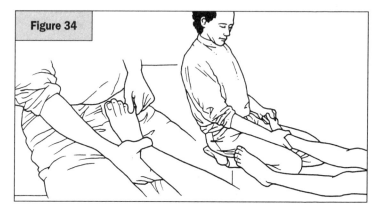

Figure 34

20. Repeat stages 16, 17, 18 and 19 on the other foot.

◆ The Hips and Legs

21. Move to the left side of the receiver, place one hand on the abdomen, and with the other hand palm down the front of the leg from the top to the ankle. Repeat on the other leg.

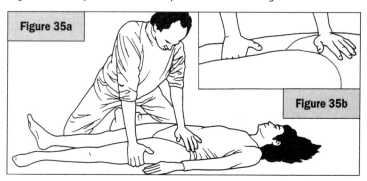

Figure 35a

Figure 35b

22. Move to between the receiver's legs, put one hand on the abdomen, and raise one leg with your other hand under the knee. Place the foot on the floor and slide your hand to the front of the knee. Raise the leg off the floor and bring the knee towards the receiver's chest. Rotate the leg, going up the inside of the body and then bringing it outwards away from the body, and down into the next rotation. Move your whole body to rotate the leg, don't just use your arm.

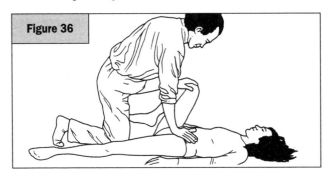

Figure 36

23. Lean on the leg, bringing the knee towards the chest, to stretch the buttock and back of the thigh. Place the foot back on the floor, slide your hand back under the knee, lift the leg and place it down on the floor again. Be careful not to let the leg drop suddenly as this could hurt the knee.

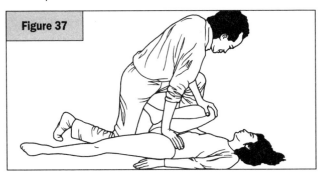

Figure 37

24. Repeat stages 22 and 23 with the other leg.

◆ The Abdomen

25. Move to a position at right-angles to the receiver's side and place both hands across the abdomen. Push into the abdomen with the heels of your hands, then pull into the abdomen with your fingers, somewhat like kneading bread. Do this ten or fifteen times.

26. Now kneel with your thigh against the receiver's. Rest your left arm on your leg and push up with the left hand under the abdomen. Use your right hand to palm in a circle around the abdomen twice, pressing twelve times at the positions of the twelve hours of a clock.

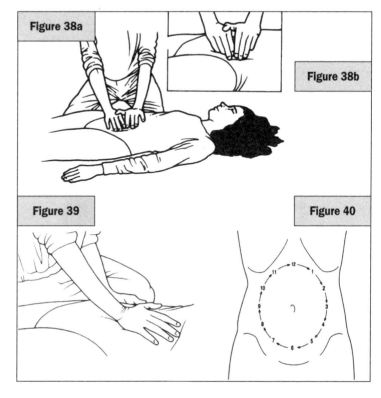

Figure 38a

Figure 38b

Figure 39

Figure 40

Now repeat, using your fingers to press more deeply. This gives deep massage to the organs of the abdomen: the stomach, small and large intestines, liver, gall bladder, pancreas and spleen. Some places may be sensitive so go gently at first.

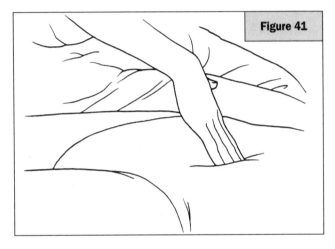

Figure 41

27. Put your right hand on the lower abdomen below the navel, push in gently and hold for ten or twenty seconds to bring Ki into the receiver's Hara.

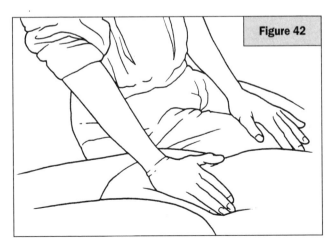

Figure 42

◆ The Chest

28. Move to the receiver's head and kneel with your knees either side of their head. All the rest of the Shiatsu treatment is given from this position. Bring each arm out to the side with the palm upwards to open the shoulder. Put the heels of your hands inside the shoulder, and lean your weight onto the shoulders. Hold for a few seconds, rock backwards, and then repeat a few more times. You may well feel the shoulders moving towards the floor as the chest opens.

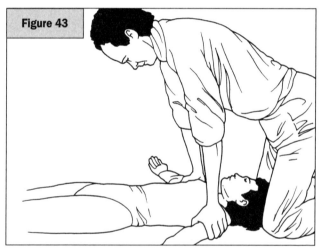

Figure 43

29. Keep one hand on the shoulder, and place the other hand on the lower ribs on the opposite side of the body. Lean forwards onto both hands, stretching the chest open. Shift your moving hand up towards the head a little and repeat. For a man you can continue to move your hand up, pressing in five or six places until the moving hand reaches the shoulder. For a woman, pressure on the breasts is uncomfortable, so bring your hand inside the breast, using the side of your hand to give pressure.

30. When your moving hand reaches the shoulder, keep it there and use your other hand to repeat stage 29 on the other side of the chest.You may well notice that the receiver's chest is now broader and more open, and that the shoulders naturally lie closer to the ground.

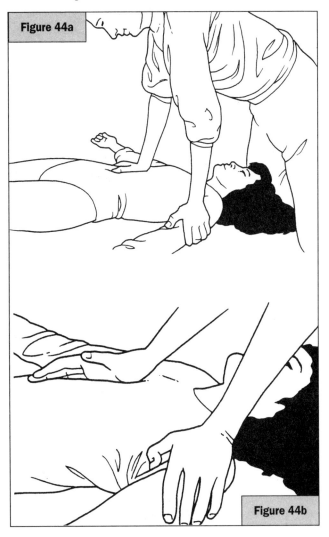

Figure 44a

Figure 44b

◆ The Arms and Hands

31. With one hand on the shoulder, palm down the length of the arm and onto the hand twice. Give lighter pressure on the elbow.

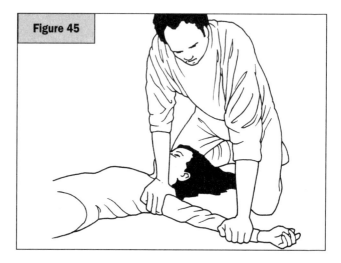

Figure 45

32. Pick up the hand, and holding the hand and wrist, lean backwards to stretch the arm and shoulder. Hold the stretch for a few seconds, release, then stretch again.

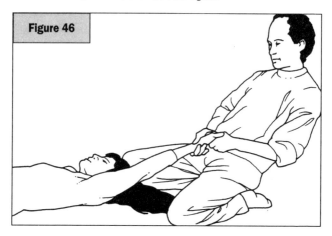

Figure 46

33. Open the palm of the hand by pressing down with the heels of your hands and upwards with your fingers. Repeat three or four times.

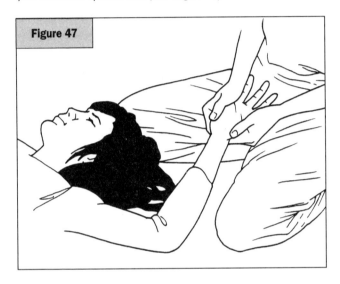

Figure 47

34. Use one thumb to press down three lines on the palm.

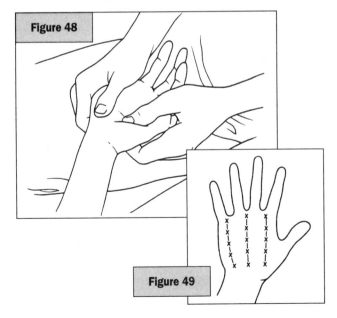

Figure 48

Figure 49

35. Grasp the hand firmly with one hand, and hold the base of the little finger with your other thumb and first finger. As with the toes, firmly rotate the finger to loosen its joint with the hand.

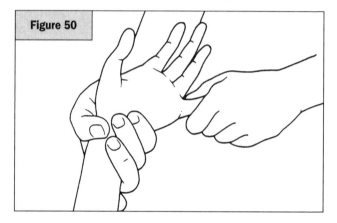

Figure 50

36. Squeeze the base of the little finger, move your fingers up a little and squeeze again. Work up to the tip of the little finger.

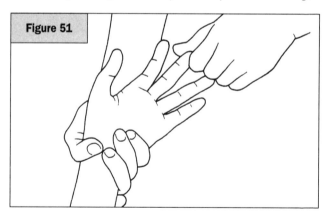

Figure 51

37. Repeat stages 35 and 36 with the other fingers and thumb.

38. Put the hand down on the floor and repeat stages 31 to 37 on the other arm and hand.

◆ The Neck

Most people carry a lot of tension in the neck, and will really enjoy Shiatsu in this area. Promoting Ki flow in the neck can help relaxation and Ki flow in the whole body.

39. Place the fingers of one hand on the spine just below the skull, and put the fingers of your other hand over the first hand's fingers. Raise the neck slightly so that the head tips backwards a little. Lean backwards to stretch the neck away from the body, with your fingers pulling on the back of the skull. Hold for a few seconds, release, then repeat. If there isn't too much tension in the neck, you will feel it lengthen, maybe by half an inch or so.

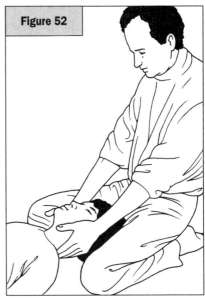

Figure 52

40. Place your hands on the sides of the head with your fingers behind the ears and your thumbs in front of the ears. Pick up the head, turn it to the side, and put it down on one hand. This hand supports the head while you work on the neck with the other hand. Use your thumb to press into the top of the neck just under the back edge of the skull. Begin just behind the ear, move half an inch towards the spine and press again. Continue until you reach the spine, where you will find a depression between the top vertebrae and the skull. Press into this depression.

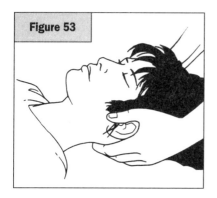

Figure 53

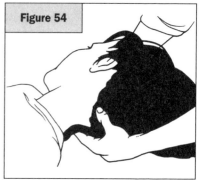

Figure 54

41. Palm the side of the head, beginning at the front and pressing in three or four places to cover the whole side of the head.

42. Put your moving hand back on the side of the head with your fingers behind the ears, pick up the head and turn it to the other side. Repeat stages 40 and 41 on the other side of the neck and head. Put your moving hand back on the side of the head, pick the head up and place it back down on the ground.

43. Put one hand under the neck and slide it under the head. Hold the neck with the other hand, and using both hands stretch the head to the side. Hold for a few seconds, then return the head to the floor. Slide your other hand under the head and do the stretch for the other side of the neck.

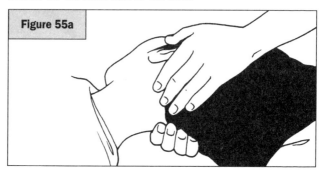

Figure 55a

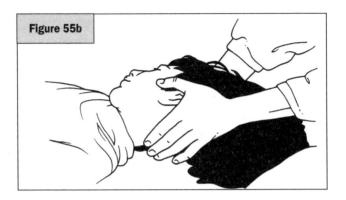

Figure 55b

44. Slide one hand under the head again, pick it up, and place your forearm behind the head with the hand on the opposite shoulder. Bring your body up so that your forearm brings the head up, stretching open the back of the neck. Hold for a few seconds, then withdraw your forearm and gently replace the head on the floor. The receiver must be fully confident that you have full control of their head and won't drop it! If there is any doubt, they will tense their neck, and your Shiatsu will have less effect.

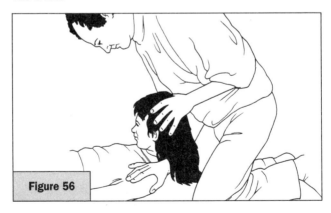

Figure 56

45. Stretch the neck as in stage 39 again. The neck will often stretch more this time as your other work has relaxed the neck.

◆ The Head and Face

46. Grip the head gently but firmly with one hand, and use the thumb of the other hand to press in a line from between the eyebrows to the top of the head, moving about half an inch each time.

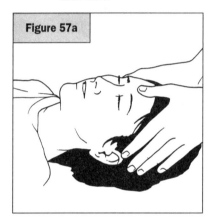

Figure 57a

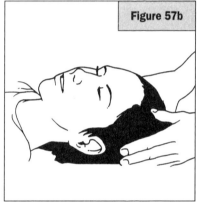

Figure 57b

47. Rest the fingers firmly on the sides of the head and use your thumbs to press in two lines from the inner edge of the eyebrows to the top of the head.

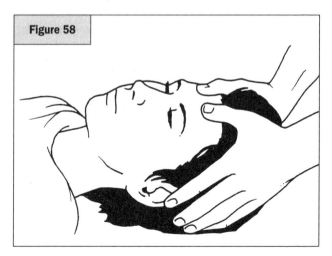

Figure 58

48. Keep your fingers firmly on the sides of the head and use both thumbs to work from the inner edge of the eyebrows across the forehead above the eyebrows to the temples.

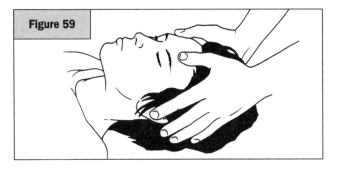

Figure 59

49. Now use your thumbs to work along the bony ridge under the eyes, moving about a quarter of an inch each time.

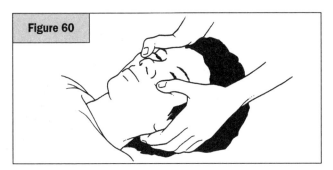

Figure 60

50. Press just to the side of the nostrils, then move in a line under the cheekbones.

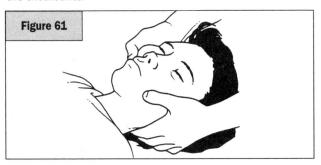

Figure 61

51. Press with one thumb between the nose and upper lip, and then with both thumbs out across the upper jaw.

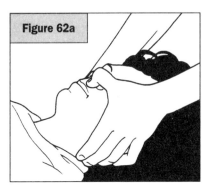

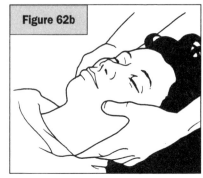

52. Press with one thumb just below the lower lip, and then with both thumbs out across the lower jaw.

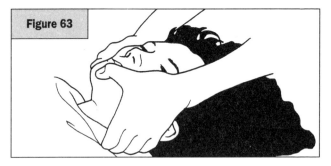

53. Place the fingers of both hands under the lower jaw and lean back to give pressure on the underside of the jaw.

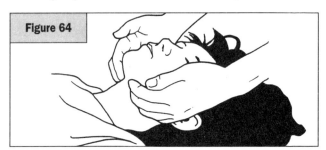

54. You have now finished your Shiatsu treatment. Place your hands lightly on either side of the head for ten or fifteen seconds, then slowly draw your hands away. Tell the receiver that you have finished, and that they should lie quietly for a few minutes until they feel ready to get up. Move to their side and sit quietly until they get up. They may well want to ask you some questions, or to share their experience of the Shiatsu with you. You may also want to ask them how the Shiatsu treatment felt to get some useful feedback.

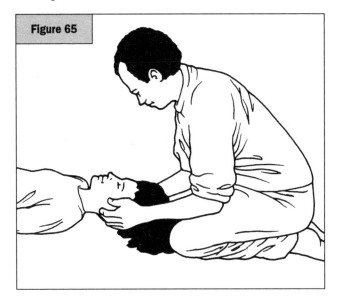

Figure 65

Congratulations! You have probably just completed your first full Shiatsu treatment. You may well be feeling that it was very complicated, and that there is an awful lot to remember. Now is the time to get some more practise in. Run through the basic Shiatsu sequence with some more friends over the next few days or weeks. You will be surprised at how easily you will remember all the actions once you have run through the full sequence a few times.

Learning to give a basic Shiatsu treatment is rather like learning to ride a bicycle – at first you have to concentrate hard on all your movements, but once you 'get the hang of it' you can stop thinking about the bicycle at all and concentrate on cycling along the road. You can start experimenting to find out just what you can do on the bicycle, as well as how to avoid cars! After giving a dozen or so Shiatsu treatments you will be able to stop thinking about yourself, and concentrate on the receiver. Then, as with riding a bicycle, Shiatsu becomes much more interesting, for you will begin noticing just how different everyone's bodies are, and how the body actually 'asks you' to vary your Shiatsu for different individuals and for different areas on one body.

The next chapter will give you some guidelines on how to adapt your Shiatsu to different individuals' needs. The following three chapters will expand your understanding of the Energetic basis of life, and will enable you to further develop and refine your Shiatsu treatments.

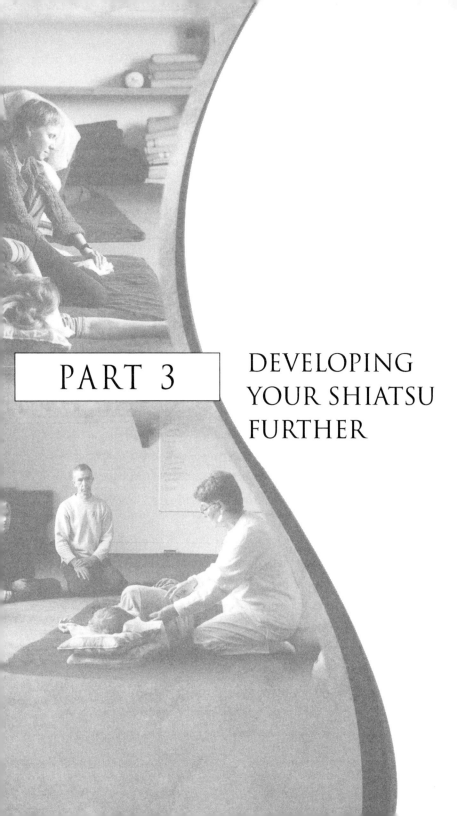

PART 3

DEVELOPING YOUR SHIATSU FURTHER

Chapter 7

ADAPTING YOUR SHIATSU FOR DIFFERENT PEOPLE

Now that you have mastered the basic Shiatsu sequence, you can concentrate more on how to vary your Shiatsu for individuals of different ages, characters, and levels of health.

You already make your own intuitive judgements about people's health and character. What you can now learn is to incorporate this judgement into your Shiatsu treatments. It can be so important to get the general approach to the whole person you are giving Shiatsu to right. You can give a technically brilliant Shiatsu treatment to someone, but unless your overall approach is appropriate it could be completely wasted. So remember, you can ask people you are giving Shiatsu to, 'How does this feel?', 'Is this too hard or too soft?', and so on.

Also remember that in Chapter 3 you did an exercise, picking up a partner who first thought of themselves as being heavy, and then as light. You will have felt a difference in their weight, merely because of their different thoughts, because we can move Energy with our minds. So in giving Shiatsu, if we are holding the thought in our mind that we want to give a sensitive, supportive, strong or vigorous Shiatsu treatment, this will make a difference to the quality of the Shiatsu we give.

A few examples of what you may perceive about people, and how to adapt your Shiatsu to their individual needs, are given below. As you give Shiatsu to more and more people you will develop your ability to adjust your approach for each person.

The Receiver	Your Treatment
Overall the person's energy seems weak, with a lack of vitality, possibly with a limp body and a lack of mental positivity	➤ Firm, supportive, nourishing Shiatsu
Overall the person's energy seems full, with an excessive amount of physical and maybe emotional energy	➤ A calming and relaxing Shiatsu
An emotionally sensitive person	➤ A gentle, sensitive Shiatsu, with care not to give too much pressure which could make them withdraw fearfully
A large, physically strong person	➤ Use more of your weight to give stronger pressure and stretches
A small, frail, elderly person	➤ Go very gently, taking care not to use too much pressure or to stretch too strongly
A healthy and active ten-year-old child	➤ Use less pressure than with an adult, and if the child is restless, give a shorter treatment
Low pain threshold	➤ Go gently!
High pain threshold, or enjoys feeling some mild pain	➤ Go more strongly

Chapter 8

THE NEXT STEP – KYO AND JITSU

The next step in developing your Shiatsu is to start using 'Kyo' and 'Jitsu'. In Shiatsu we are primarily working with Energy. Obviously the amount or intensity of Energy in different people and in different parts of the body is very basic to our working with Energy. Kyo and Jitsu are used to describe the states of deficient or low Energy (*Kyo*) and excess or high Energy (*Jitsu*).

Kyo and Jitsu can be used at different levels, from considering the amount of Energy in a whole person, in different areas of the body, in the Meridians, and at specific Tsubos.

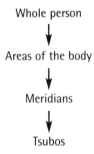

Whole person
↓
Areas of the body
↓
Meridians
↓
Tsubos

Students beginning to learn Shiatsu generally find it easier to diagnose Kyo and Jitsu on the broader levels of the whole person and in areas of the body. As you study Shiatsu further, you will progress to perceiving Meridians and Tsubos through touch and visually, and will then be able to diagnose Kyo and Jitsu in the Meridians and Tsubos.

◆ Diagnosis of Kyo and Jitsu

It is relatively easy to tell whether the whole person is more Kyo or Jitsu. If someone is low in physical energy, with a rather limp looking body without much muscle tone, and maybe a rather negative or depressed emotional or mental expression, they could be said to be more Kyo. They will probably give the feeling of needing support and nourishment. So the overall direction of your Shiatsu needs to be firm, supportive and energizing. A person who is lively, active, and expressive with high muscle tone could be described as being more Jitsu. They may give the feeling of needing to stop and relax for once. So you can make your Shiatsu more calming and relaxing, for example by going slowly without sudden movements.

Kyo and Jitsu also exists in different areas of the body. In Chapter 2 we saw that our life and health depends on the flow of Energy through the body, and that ideally Energy should be more or less evenly distributed in different Chakras, Organs, and Meridians. Nobody ever achieves a perfect balance, but we can all work to improve the balance of Energy in different parts of the body for increased health. One way of doing this is through Shiatsu. As one becomes more practised in giving Shiatsu, one begins to pick up on areas of the body where the Energy is low, and others where the Energy is high.

Kyo and Jitsu can be diagnosed visually by looking at a person, from touching a person during a Shiatsu treatment, and by the receiver's response to your touch. Before giving a Shiatsu you may see imbalances, which give a general guide as to which parts of the body need some extra attention. Then, during the Shiatsu, through your touch you will pick up on Kyo and Jitsu areas in greater detail. Also, while giving Shiatsu, if you are perceptive about how the person is feeling, you can pick up on their response. Of course they

may also tell you how your Shiatsu feels. So giving Shiatsu is quite
a curious blend of both diagnosis and treatment.

Visually, if you quickly scan your eyes over another person, your
attention will be drawn to certain places, for example the legs,
hands, knees, or part of the back. These areas are usually those
which are out of balance. The body could be described as
consisting of 'mountains' where areas stand out, due to an excess
of Ki, and 'valleys' where areas appear hollow or weak, because of
a deficiency of Ki. If a person is in relatively good health there are
relatively few mountains and valleys, and these are not so marked.
If the valleys and mountains are more marked, then the person's Ki
is more imbalanced, and their health is probably poorer.

	Kyo	Jitsu
Visual Diagnosis	Area is hollow or depressed	Area is raised, standing out
	Weak looking with a lack of muscle tension	Excess muscle tension
Touch Diagnosis	Feels unnaturally soft (or with surface tension, with weakness beneath)	Feels hard
	May feel cold	May feel hot
	Feels empty or lifeless	Feels full and alive
	Feels needy, asking to be held	Feels repelling, not wanting to be touched
	Difficult to find, hidden	Usually easy to find, obvious
Receiver's Response	Feels vulnerable	Feels safe
	Deep, unpleasant pain	Local discomfort or pain
	Deep relaxation and nourishment	Local relaxation and relief

As you become more practised in giving Shiatsu you will probably naturally begin noticing that some parts of your friends' bodies feel hard and tense, while other areas feel soft, with a lack of muscle tone, and an empty or lifeless feeling. These are physical signs that the areas are Jitsu or Kyo. When a place is greatly depleted in Energy, that is it is very Kyo, a stiff surface tension may develop, hiding the underlying Kyo. As you give Shiatsu to such an area, the surface tension will usually relax, revealing the weakness below. At some point in your learning of Shiatsu you will also come to sense Ki directly, as in the first two exercises you practised in Chapter 3. As this sense of Ki becomes more definite it can be used as the main way of diagnosing Kyo and Jitsu during your Shiatsu.

Thirdly, Kyo and Jitsu can be identified by the sensations of the person receiving your Shiatsu. Kyo places are weak, and so vulnerable. If pressure is given too suddenly or too hard, a person experiences deep unpleasant pain, and feels invaded or attacked. Their body may recoil to protect this place of weakness. On the other hand if gentle, sensitive, firm and supportive pressure is given, the person deeply relaxes, and feels great relief and nourishment from the Shiatsu. Appropriate Shiatsu on Kyo areas, Meridians or Tsubos brings deep relaxation and healing to the whole person.

If too much pressure is given on a Jitsu place, it may feel uncomfortable, but only in that localized area and not throughout the body. It is more bearable than too much pressure on a Kyo place. Appropriate Shiatsu on Jitsu places creates relaxation more at the surface and at just that location, and does not have such a deep or wide effect as Shiatsu on a Kyo place.

◆ Treating Kyo and Jitsu

From what has been said above, you can see that varying your
Shiatsu according to Kyo and Jitsu will increase the effectiveness of
your Shiatsu. When you follow the basic Shiatsu sequence
described in the last chapter you will actually tend to rebalance
both Kyo and Jitsu areas. Both pressure with the palms or thumbs
and stretches will generally tend to bring Kyo and Jitsu places back
into balance. However, as you become more conscious of Kyo and
Jitsu within the body, your Shiatsu can become more specific, and
so more beneficial. Some general guidelines can be given on how
to vary your Shiatsu according to Kyo and Jitsu. These are not rigid
rules, but just pointers to help you develop your own sense of what
is appropriate to do for different people and on different parts of
the body.

Kyo	Jitsu
A sensitive touch is needed	Use pressure with the palms or thumbs for a shorter time to move the excess Energy out of the area
Hold pressure with the palm or thumb for a longer time, for ten or fifteen seconds or until you feel the place has come alive	
	Stretching for a short time can be very effective at moving the Energy out of Jitsu areas
Stretches can be held for longer to bring Energy into an area	
	Movements like rocking and shaking parts of the body can help move excess Energy out of an area

Don't get too intellectual in using Kyo and Jitsu; for example, getting in a panic because you can't identify Kyo and Jitsu areas in a particular person. Rather, as you 'tune into' the bodies of the people you are giving Shiatsu to, Kyo and Jitsu will 'appear' to you. You can then change your approach according to what you see or feel, either holding a Kyo area or Tsubo longer, or working to dispel the Energy from a Jitsu area or Tsubo.

When beginning to look for Kyo and Jitsu within the body, Jitsu places often stand out more than Kyo places. It can then be tempting to work more on these Jitsu places, trying to dispel the excess tension and Energy. However this way of working will only have a more superficial effect, unless Kyo places are also identified and treated appropriately. It is generally most effective to work on both Kyo and Jitsu places within a full-body Shiatsu treatment, and not just concentrate on either one of these imbalances.

If someone has pain in a particular part of their body, the Energy in that place is always either Kyo or Jitsu. Pain caused by an area being Kyo is generally of the chronic, nagging, dull, deep kind. Pain caused by an area being Jitsu is usually more of the acute, intense or stabbing kind. If you can rebalance the Energy in painful areas, the pain will almost always go. If the person has had the pain for a long time, then several treatments may be needed to rebalance the Energy and remove the pain.

It takes dozens or hundreds of Shiatsu treatments to really get the hang of perceiving and working with Kyo and Jitsu. It is a gradual process of learning to perceive Ki more clearly. Regular practise is the key to a better understanding, as in learning any practical skill. So now that you are gaining in confidence in giving healing Shiatsu treatments, find some more friends or willing members of your family to keep practising on.

Chapter 9

THE ENERGETICS
OF FOOD

Oriental medicine uses several approaches to balance Energy in the body, and so promote health or alleviate illness. Having examined one approach, Shiatsu, we are going to briefly look at another, the use of diet. As well as giving Shiatsu treatments, Shiatsu practitioners frequently give clients advice on steps that they can take themselves to promote their health, such as advising changes in diet and activity, and practising specific exercises. These kinds of lifestyle changes complement Shiatsu treatment very well, and can greatly add to the health benefits. As with other aspects of Oriental medicine, food is considered mainly in Energetic terms. I think you will find this approach very interesting and revealing.

At present the common way of looking at food is based on the scientific analysis of foods into its constituents – carbohydrates, fats, protein, vitamins, minerals and fibre. This approach is useful in ensuring that we get enough of the various nutrients that our bodies need, such as vitamins, minerals and essential amino acids, and that we do not over-consume certain nutrients like fats or simple sugars. However, this modern nutritional theory alone does not ensure good health; one may be eating enough of the various nutrients our bodies need, and still get ill. It also gives little indication of the emotional, psychological and spiritual effects of different foods.

Our understanding of the relationship between food and health can be greatly extended by looking at the Energetic qualities of the foods we eat. Just as the body has traditionally been regarded Energetically, food can also be understood in terms of Energy. One can then understand how foods interact and change the Energetic constitution of the body. It can give an exact method of comprehending the effects of particular foods on us physically, emotionally, mentally and spiritually.

Furthermore, a knowledge of the Energetic nature of the body and of foods, combined with methods of Oriental diagnosis for ascertaining the condition of the various Organs and systems of the body, enables one to work out exactly which foods are most harmful and most beneficial for a particular individual. This approach can be used by anyone to improve their health and steadily reduce the chances of their suffering from illness in the future, as well as for alleviating a very wide range of health problems.

This chapter gives a brief introduction to this approach to understanding the Energetics of foods and their effects on our health, with broad recommendations on how to eat a healthier diet. The next chapter, on Oriental diagnosis, will give you a more precise idea of how particular foods may have contributed to health problems, and of beneficial dietary changes that can be made to alleviate them.

◆ Yin and Yang

In considering food as Energy, we need a way of describing Energy. The most useful way is to use Yin and Yang, which describe the direction of the movement of Energy. (This is different to Kyo and Jitsu, which describe the intensity of Energy.) Traditionally it was considered that the two fundamental directions of movement are expansion and contraction, and that the interplay between these two create all forms and events in nature and the universe. Therefore everything can be described in terms of Yin and Yang.

This may seem very simplistic, and in a way it is, but its simplicity is its strength. Using Yin and Yang can help us see the essential or most basic qualities of life. Also, as everything can be described in terms of Yin and Yang, we can understand the inter-relationship of any two aspects of life or nature, such as the influence of our food on our physical health, moods and emotions and spiritual awareness, how we can adjust our food when living in different climates or seasons, and according to particular kinds of activity.

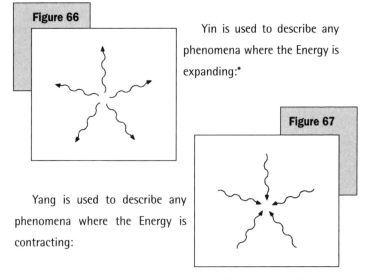

Figure 66

Yin is used to describe any phenomena where the Energy is expanding:*

Figure 67

Yang is used to describe any phenomena where the Energy is contracting:

We use many pairs of opposite qualities to describe and understand our lives – hot and cold, day and night, male and female, extrovert and introvert, rich and poor, happy and sad, young and old, to name a few. The table opposite gives some other examples of Yin and Yang.

*Here I have used the definitions found in macrobiotic teachings, as most books dealing with the Energetic qualities of food are from this source. If you have already studied Yin and Yang in Chinese philosophy and medicine, you will find that these definitions differ from the traditional definitions. George Ohsawa, who began teaching macrobiotics, changed the traditional view that Yang is expansion and Yin is contraction to Yang symbolizing contraction and Yin symbolizing expansion, thinking that this system would be more easily understood by people in the West. This was the only change he made; other qualities such as hot and cold, night and day, and active and passive remained the same as in the traditional definition.

This change of definition should present no great problem for students of Oriental philosophy and medicine. The words 'Yin' and 'Yang' are quite arbitrary – different words could be used, or the classification of Yin phenomena and Yang phenomena could be reversed. The only important thing, as with all language, is that their basic definition is clearly stated so that a word can carry meaning to another person. However Yin and Yang are defined, the universal symmetry of nature remains unchanged and eternal.

	Yang	Yin
Movement	Contraction	Expansion
Natural Cycles	Day	Night
	Summer	Winter
	Activity	Rest
	Work	Play
	Tension	Relaxation
	Growth	Decay
	Life	Death
Air	Carbon Dioxide	Oxygen
	Hotter	Colder
	Dryer	Wetter
	Positive ions	Negative ions
Vibrations	Longer waves	Shorter waves
	Red - Orange - Yellow - Green - Blue - Violet	
	Radio waves	X-rays
The Body	Male sex	Female sex
	Solid organs e.g. liver	Hollow organs e.g. stomach
	Parasympathetic nervous system	Sympathetic nervous system
	Inbreath	Outbreath
	Physical and social activity	Mental and spiritual activity
Dimension	Time	Space

◆ The Yin and Yang of Food

When we look at our food in terms of Yin and Yang, the most fundamental division we can make is between animal and plant foods. Using the pairs of qualities given above we can work out whether animals or plants are more Yin or Yang. Animals are active, contain red blood, are often warm-blooded, and are concentrated in that they eat many times their bodyweight to create their bodies. The Energetic nature of animals can therefore be said to be Yang. Plants, on the other hand, are passive, are based on the colour green of chlorophyll, and are generally cool. Plants have a more expanded form, with many leaves and numerous roots in the soil, whereas the body of animals is compact with their 'leaves' internally in the lungs and their 'roots' along the length of the intestines. Plants have a more expansive, or Yin, Energetic nature.

We can also distinguish a third major category of foods. Many foods are created from various extracts from plants, such as sugar, oil, stimulants like coffee and tea, spices, and alcohol. These extracts are nearly always a more Yin or expansive part of the plants, so this group of foods is more expansive or Yin than the plants they come from.

We now have three broad groups of foods, as shown in the table opposite.

Salt is not a living food, but a mineral, and is very contractive, and so is placed in the Yang category.

Milk has a more expansive nature. The Energetic nature of foods made from milk varies according to how they are made; hard cheeses are harder and more condensed, and are generally quite salty, and so are more Yang. Yoghurt and cream are lighter and have a more expansive Energy than milk.

Yang Foods	Balanced Foods	Yin Foods
meat	cereal grains	oil
eggs	vegetables	fruit juices
poultry	beans	sugar
fish	seeds	honey
seafood	nuts	stimulants
cheese	temperate fruits	alcohol
salt	sea vegetables	milk
miso		yoghurt
		cream
		spices
		most drugs e.g. aspirin, cortisone
		refined foods
		most chemical food additives
		tropical fruits and vegetables

Foods that grow in a hotter tropical climate (Yang) are generally more expanded or Yin. Tropical fruits like oranges, pineapples and dates, and vegetables of a tropical origin, including potatoes, tomatoes, peppers and aubergines, therefore fall into the Yin category.

As we have seen, everything in our world and lives is created by Yin and Yang. These two forces nourish and sustain our whole being – the body, emotions, mind and spirit. At a physical level the balance between Yin and Yang has a very profound effect on our health, such as the all important sodium-potassium and acid-alkaline balance of the blood and body, the production of hormones with opposite effects such as insulin and glycogon or oestrogen and progesterone, the expansion and contraction of organs like the heart, lungs and intestines, and in the two halves of the autonomic nervous system – the sympathetic and parasympathetic – which are basic to the smooth functioning of the entire body.

We experience the Yang force as creating inner strength and warmth, energy and vitality, tension, and the ability to be busy or working. The Yin force takes Energy outwards in the body to be used in our physical movement, actions and expression. It also has a cooling effect, and creates more relaxation.

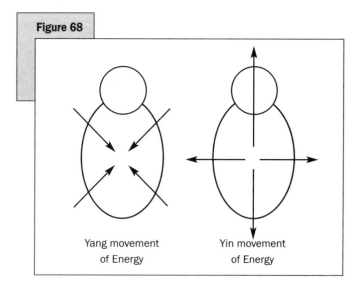

Figure 68

Yang movement
of Energy

Yin movement
of Energy

Looking at this figure you can imagine how emotionally the Yang force produces more centredness, groundedness, stability, constancy and reliability, whereas the Yin force produces more expressiveness, creativity, communication and sociability.

Mentally, the Yang movement produces greater focus or concentration, more analytical and intellectual thinking, while the Yin movement produces more artistic, imaginative and creative thinking, with a broader or wholistic perspective.

When these two forces are in balance we experience health in body and mind. In this view health can be defined as 'a balance between Yin and Yang in our physical, emotional, mental and spiritual being'. This can be illustrated as:

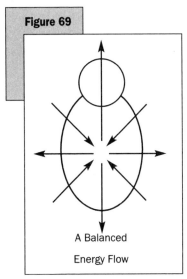

Figure 69

A Balanced

Energy Flow

Thinking of health in terms of Yin and Yang is also more useful as it relates to our common everyday experience. We often talk about our Energy being 'high' or 'low', elated or depressed, inwardly-turned (introverted) or outwardly-turned (extroverted). Sometimes we feel 'stuck' or 'blocked' when the flow of Energy through the body is just that, and 'out of sorts' or 'off-balance' when it is imbalanced. When our Energy flow is smooth and unimpeded we feel happy, and when the Energy flow is poor we feel sadness.

◆ A Diet of Extremes

There are many influences in our lives that affect the balance of Yin and Yang Energy within us, but our food is undoubtedly one of the most fundamental factors affecting our Energy balance. We eat several times a day, day-in day-out, for all of our lives. If we look at the typical modern diet in terms of Yin and Yang we can see that it is predominantly made up of the more extreme Yin and extreme Yang foods, as shown on the following page. When we look at this figure it is really not surprising that in modern society we suffer from such a multitude of physical illnesses and psychological problems resulting from an imbalanced state of health.

Although people are generally eating both the extreme Yin and Yang foods, many people eat proportionately more of the Yang foods, or more of the Yin foods. Therefore problems can be caused by one of three ways of imbalanced eating – predominantly extreme Yang foods, extreme Yin foods, or a combination of both. The Energy movement in each case is illustrated below:

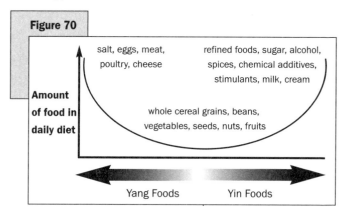

Figure 70

Amount of food in daily diet

salt, eggs, meat, poultry, cheese

refined foods, sugar, alcohol, spices, chemical additives, stimulants, milk, cream

whole cereal grains, beans, vegetables, seeds, nuts, fruits

Yang Foods   Yin Foods

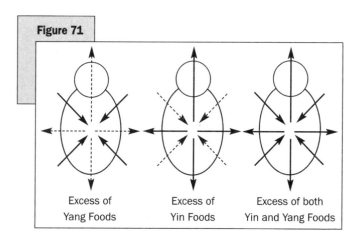

Figure 71

Excess of Yang Foods   Excess of Yin Foods   Excess of both Yin and Yang Foods

In the first case, when large amounts of Yang foods like meat, eggs and salt are eaten, various parts of the body become contracted, hardened and stiffened. For example, a diet high in animal fats is well known to create arteriosclerosis in which the walls of the arteries become thickened and hardened.

It is easy to see that an excess of Yang foods will cause a build up of Energy deep inside the body. This is experienced as deep tension and the feeling of being bottled up. These people can appear 'uptight', and often keep a tight control over their emotions and life, repressing their feelings and reacting to situations logically and intellectually. The bottled-up Energy sometimes escapes in bursts, causing outbursts of anger, impatience and frustration. There is a tendency to become more rigid, stubborn and inflexible. Such people often hold on tightly to their views or way of life, denying the ideas of others and resisting any changes in their lives. Think of your friends and acquaintances and you will probably be able to identify some that have these characteristics.

When a person has eaten large amounts of the more extreme Yin foods such as sugar, sweets and other foods high in sugar, honey, spices and tropical vegetables and fruits, the body's organs become expanded, enlarged and weakened. Enlargement of the heart can cause poor circulation, and eventually heart problems. Expansion of the intestines is very common, causing irregular bowel movements with either diarrhoea or constipation, and more severe problems like colitis.

Consuming more of the extreme Yin foods moves Energy to the surface of the body. This can create more surface tension or nervousness, anxiety, over-excitability and over-emotional behaviour. At the same time the Energy deep inside the body becomes depleted, causing an inner weakness that may be expressed as fearfulness, worry, under-confidence or stress. Thinking tends to become vague or 'spaced out'. There may be difficulty in maintaining concentration in work or in any pursuit, and a tendency to give up on things before they are completed. Money and opportunities 'slip through the hands' all too easily. Again, think through people you know and you will probably be able to think of some with these qualities.

A diet with approximately equal amounts of the more extreme Yin and extreme Yang foods brings about a variety of health problems involving contraction and expansion, such as formation of stones in the kidneys and gall bladder, many skin ailments, and breast cysts and tumours. This combination of both extremes also creates a mixture of the emotions and thinking described above. Often there are swings in mood from one extreme to the other, such as from fear to anger, or depression to aggression.

◆ Traditional Diets from Around the World

It is informative to look at the traditional diets of peoples from around the world because they often arrived at a relatively healthy way of eating through trial and error over hundreds or thousands of years. This way of eating sustained them over many generations. Much of this traditional wisdom has been lost in the modern world of mass-produced and convenience foods. We must be careful not to idealize any traditional way of eating as the ideal way, as most ancient cultures still suffered from illness, and were often constrained by the limited range of foods available locally. However, many of today's diseases, especially of the serious degenerative illnesses like cancer, diabetes and heart disease, were absent or little known in many traditional cultures.

A brief look at traditional diets from around the world reveals a consistent pattern of eating. Broadly speaking we can see two major dietary patterns. Firstly, peoples living in the far north of Asia and America, such as in Siberia, northern Scandinavia, Greenland and northern Canada, relied heavily on animal foods, as these were the main food available to them. Judging by reports on the health of the Eskimos and other inhabitants of the far north, this diet was relatively healthy. In such an extreme cold climate with plenty of physical activity, a high animal fat diet seems necessary to provide the body heat and energy necessary for survival. This would be expected from using the theory of Yin and Yang – living in a colder or Yin climate, a more Yang diet is necessary to keep in balance with the environment. Unless we are living under similar conditions, this can hardly be considered a sensible way for us to eat.

The second major dietary pattern can be seen in peoples living in temperate and tropical climates. Some kind of whole cereal grain has usually formed the largest part of the diet with a smaller amount of beans. Fresh vegetables were eaten in fairly large quantities where available, mostly cooked, with some eaten raw. A little fish, dairy, meat, or certain fermented foods such as miso, tempeh and shoyu soy sauce made from soya beans were used, with pickled vegetables like sauerkraut, and fermented drinks like beer and wine. This last group of animal foods and fermented foods may well have been included as a source of vitamin B12, which is not generally present in fresh plant foods. Fruits were generally eaten in small quantities. This major dietary pattern is illustrated in Figure 72.

While many major cultures' diet followed this basic pattern, the specific types of foods used in each category varied greatly depending on the kinds of food plants that grew well locally.

In India the main part of the meal was usually bread or rice, with a smaller amount of dahl made from beans or peas, a dish of cooked vegetables, and a small serving of yoghurt, fish or fowl. Often a little fruit or raw food like sprouted beans or salad greens was also added.

Figure 72

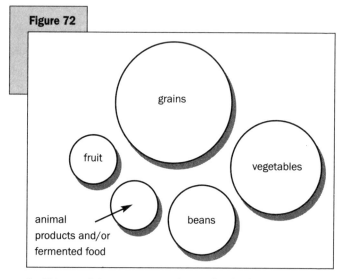

In China and Japan most meals consisted of rice and cooked vegetables with smaller amounts of beans, fish, meat or fermented soya bean products. In parts of China rice was replaced with millet or wheat.

North American Indians were mainly hunters and gatherers, but in the south agriculture was practised. Corn, cornbread or tortillas comprised the largest part of a meal, with smaller amounts of leafy green vegetables, beans and peas, and occasionally meat, dairy or fish.

The Middle Eastern diet is primarily based on a flat bread (pita) and garbanzo beans (chickpeas) with some cooked vegetables and yoghurt, fish or meat.

These traditional diets still form the basic way of eating for a large part of the world's population. In northern Europe it is more difficult to discover people's traditional eating patterns, as this region has been most affected by industrialization and the development of many refined and artificial factory-made foods. However, bread made from wheat, barley or rye seems to be found everywhere, with pasta or noodles prevalent in some Mediterranean countries, and these probably formed the largest part of the diet. Various kinds of beans and peas were eaten in most areas, although this tradition has now been lost in many parts. Locally available vegetables were eaten, and some dairy, fish or meat formed a smaller part of the diet. In addition, fermented drinks like beer and wine seem to have been standard fare.

From this brief survey of dietary patterns from around the world, we can see that the diet of most stable groups of peoples in temperate and tropical climates have been primarily made up of foods in the Energetically balanced group. Is this a mere coincidence? With the extremely wide range of foods available this can hardly have occurred by chance. Through simple trial and error over many generations this was most probably found to be the most economical and healthy way of eating.

As we have seen, our modern way of eating is practically opposite to this traditional balanced Yin-Yang dietary pattern. When we have been raised on this modern diet of meat, dairy, sugar and refined grains it seems like the normal way to eat, but in view of the diets eaten by humankind over thousands of years around the world, it can be seen to be a very recent and localized experiment in eating. By all accounts, it is rather a failure! It has brought ever-increasing poor health and disease, as well as the widespread destruction of our soil and environment.

◆ Eating a Balanced Diet

Choosing our food mainly from the Energetically balanced group will, over time, greatly enhance the creation of a balance in Energy in the different subtle bodies, Chakras, Organs and Meridians, and therefore also in the physical body. This balanced way of eating is shown below.

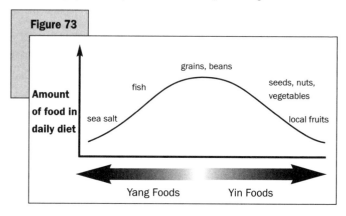

Figure 73

Amount of food in daily diet — sea salt, fish, grains, beans, seeds, nuts, vegetables, local fruits — Yang Foods / Yin Foods

For example, eating a lot of animal foods in the more Yang food group over-energises the lower Chakras. This tends to make people more assertive and individualistic. This way of eating has actually contributed much to the whole mentality and civilization of modern Western society. When large amounts of the more Yin food group are regularly eaten, the lower Chakras become weak, and the upper Chakras are over-stimulated. This can make people ungrounded and impractical, and overly preoccupied with mental and spiritual activities. Eating a diet based on the balanced group of foods will create a balance in the activity of the different Chakras, which will be reflected in greater balance in the physical, emotional, mental and spiritual aspects of our daily lives.

Likewise, primarily eating from the balanced food group will create a chemical and Energetic balance in the blood, body fluids and cells of the body, and in the Organs, nervous and hormonal systems. As the

116

internal Organs of the body are intimately connected to the Meridians that pass out from them over the body, an Energetic balance in the Organs will tend to create a balanced flow of Energy in the Meridians.

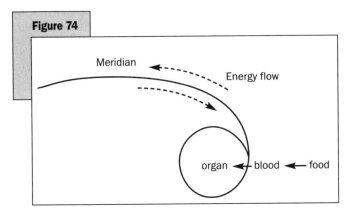

Figure 74

To understand in more practical detail how to eat from the balanced food group it is helpful to expand the three food groups into a more accurate continuous scale from the most Yang foods to the most Yin, as shown in Figure 75. Note that there is a good correlation between the Yin-Yang Energetic nature of foods and their sodium-potassium balance.

About 80 per cent of this balanced diet is made up of a variety of different whole cereal grains, beans and bean products like tofu and tempeh, and vegetables. Seeds, nuts, fruit and fish and/or fermented foods make up another 10 to 15 per cent. In addition, various seasonings are needed, such as a little sea salt, vegetable oil, shoyu soy sauce, vinegar, garlic, root ginger, herbs, and grain sweeteners like barley malt and rice syrup. Plus one needs some non-stimulating beverages like Three Year Twig Tea (also called Bancha or Kukicha), grain coffees like Barleycup, Caro and Yannoh, mild herb teas, or dandelion coffee. A little alcohol and fruit or vegetable juice can also be drunk.

There is not enough space in a book of this size to go into greater detail on eating a balanced diet. However, several books are

given in the Further Reading section that give much more
information on the Energetic nature of foods, and how to cook
balanced and varied meals.

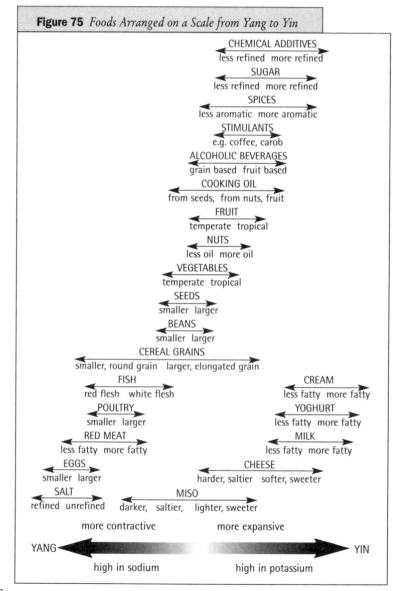

Figure 75 *Foods Arranged on a Scale from Yang to Yin*

Chapter 10

ORIENTAL DIAGNOSIS AND BODY READING

From practising the guidelines in Chapter 7, Adapting your Shiatsu for Different People, you should be getting the feel of the overall direction of your Shiatsu treatments. From Chapter 8 on Kyo and Jitsu, you may now sometimes be picking up on areas of the body where a person's Ki is more imbalanced, and in need of some extra Shiatsu. Chapter 9 outlined the influence that diet has on health. This chapter will now give you a lot of extra information on what you can learn about a person by looking at and touching them, and how you can adapt your Shiatsu according to what you observe.

The likely dietary causes of particular imbalances and problems are also given, with guidelines on beneficial changes in diet. It should be remembered that the balanced diet plan described in the last chapter is the most fundamental way of using the Energies of food to establish Energetic balance and health in the body, and should form the basis of moves to improve one's diet.

Shiatsu and dietary changes work very well together. The Shiatsu has a more immediate effect, rebalancing and stimulating the movement of a person's Ki, while changes in eating patterns have a more long-term effect, bringing about deep changes in a person's health.

By looking at the body, we can learn a great deal about the inner health of the body and a person's emotional and mental make-up. We all actually do this intuitively when we meet and interact with other people, but very often we are quite unconscious of how we do it. For example, when we first meet someone, within a second or two we may feel drawn to or repelled by them. How we greet them and what we first say to them depends on our very rapid initial assessment of the kind of person they are. Or when we see a friend, even before speaking with them we may say, 'What's getting you down today?' or 'What are you worried about?' or 'You are looking happy today'.

By studying traditional methods of Oriental diagnosis and some more modern methods of body reading, we can greatly increase the amount we can learn by simply looking at a person. Many methods of diagnosis were developed in countries like China and Japan, based on seeing, hearing, smelling, questioning and touching another person (or ourselves). These methods reveal much about a person's ancestors, parents and personality, their past environment and diet, and the present state of health of Organs and systems within the body. In this chapter we will concentrate on postural diagnosis, in which one sees or feels imbalances in the physical structure of the body, and in the distribution of Energy over the body. These methods are of direct practical use in giving Shiatsu. Recently some Western people have evolved methods of body reading that reveal much about a person's emotional and mental make-up. This approach can be used to help people on an emotional and mental level through work on the body.

Modern Western thinking has tended to focus on the physical structure of the body such as the bones, muscles, organs, skin, and so on. As we saw in Chapter 2, we are actually multi-dimensional. We have a physical body, and closely associated with it the etheric Energetic body. Then there is the astral body which relates to a person's emotions, and the mental and causal bodies. All of these bodies lie over each other, although they extend outwards to different distances.

So when we look at a particular part of the physical body, say a foot, what we see is the result of what is happening in the whole of the person's physical health, and emotional, mental and spiritual states. This can make feet very interesting! And if someone has a problem with their feet, the main cause may be in their inner physical health, in unconstructive or Energy-blocking emotions or mental beliefs, or in impediments in their spiritual evolution.

You can demonstrate this inter-relationship by standing in front of a mirror with your feet firmly on the floor, and straightening your spine and neck, and bringing your shoulders back so that your back is flat. You may find that you need to take some extra deep breaths of air, or that your breathing deepens. You may also feel more self-esteem, stronger, more open, and thoughts may enter your mind, like how you can be more effective in your life. So by changing your physical body, other changes have happened on a physical, emotional and mental level. Shiatsu primarily affects the etheric body, and through this brings about physical, emotional and mental changes.

◆ The Back and Front of the Body

In some people the back and front of the body appear quite different, with one stronger than the other, and possibly presenting a quite different character. Physically the back of the body particularly reflects the strength of the Energy in the Kidneys and Bladder, as these Meridians run mainly over the back of the body. If this Energy is strong, a person usually has 'spine', that is

Figure 76 *Diagnostic Areas on the Body - Front View*

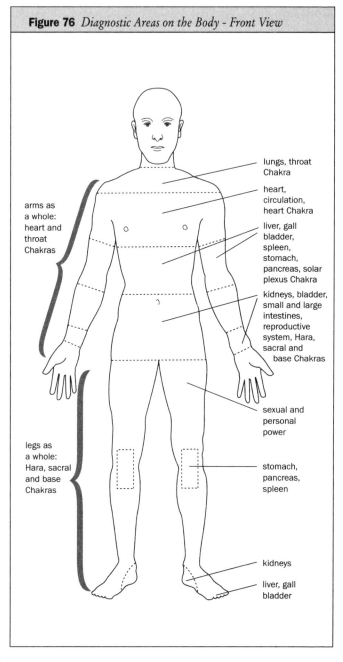

arms as
a whole:
heart and
throat
Chakras

lungs, throat
Chakra

heart,
circulation,
heart Chakra

liver, gall
bladder,
spleen,
stomach,
pancreas, solar
plexus Chakra

kidneys, bladder,
small and large
intestines,
reproductive
system, Hara,
sacral and
base Chakras

sexual and
personal
power

legs as
a whole:
Hara, sacral
and base
Chakras

stomach,
pancreas,
spleen

kidneys

liver, gall
bladder

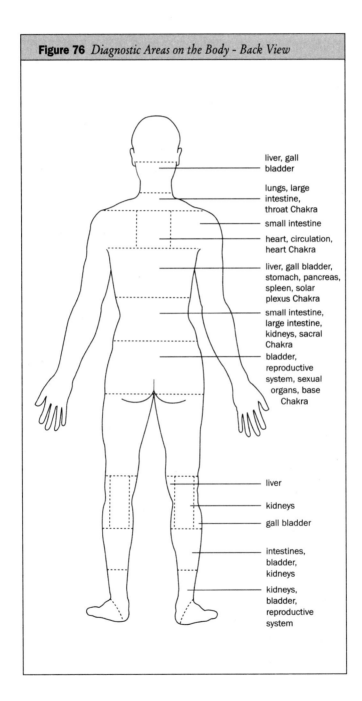

Figure 76 *Diagnostic Areas on the Body - Back View*

liver, gall bladder

lungs, large intestine, throat Chakra

small intestine

heart, circulation, heart Chakra

liver, gall bladder, stomach, pancreas, spleen, solar plexus Chakra

small intestine, large intestine, kidneys, sacral Chakra

bladder, reproductive system, sexual organs, base Chakra

liver

kidneys

gall bladder

intestines, bladder, kidneys

kidneys, bladder, reproductive system

they have courage and initiative in standing up for themselves and for what they want or think is right. If the back appears weak, a person is likely to be weak-willed, anxious and cautious. They will probably greatly enjoy strong, supportive Shiatsu down the back of their body, giving them a greater sense of inner strength and resource. They could also reduce foods that weaken the Kidneys, especially sugar, spices, tropical fruits and vegetables, excess fluid and cold foods like ice cream, and eat more foods that strengthen the Kidneys like whole cereal grains, beans (especially aduki beans), sea vegetables, and soups seasoned with barley miso. Kidney Energy is also weakened by overwork, a lack of sleep, and an excessive amount of sex, so more sleep and rest can also help.

Emotionally and mentally the back of the body reflects our unconscious. Very often there is a lot of tension in the back as a result of feelings and thoughts that have been pushed into the back of our minds. Frequently, releasing this tension with Shiatsu relieves people of a lot of negativity, leaving them feeling lighter and happier. Eating a lot of Yang foods like meat, eggs, cheese and salt also creates a lot of tension in the back, and therefore also contributes to the holding on of old emotions and thoughts. Reducing these foods and eating a more Energetically balanced diet will help to reduce tension in the back and back of the neck.

The front of the body reflects the strength of the Energy in the Stomach, Spleen and Pancreas. The Stomach and Pancreas are primarily digestive organs, but in a wider sense the Stomach and Spleen Energy determines our appetite for food and life, and how we take in and give out on a physical, emotional and mental level. If the front of the body appears weak, a person's digestive abilities may be weak, and their appetite for life and forward movement through life may be low. Eating a lot of sweets and sweet foods frequently contributes to a weakening of the Stomach and Pancreas. Replacing these foods sweetened with sugar with naturally sweet foods like onions, parsnips, squash, and dried fruits will help.

If the front of the body is strong, a person's appetite for food and for new experiences is generally strong. If there is a lot of tension in the front of the body, say in the chest, abdomen and front of the thighs, this appetite may be excessive. A person may then be restless, always in a hurry and busy. Relaxing this tension can help a person to become calmer.

◆ The Top and Bottom of the Body

There is also often an imbalance between the top of the body above the waist, and the bottom of the body. The strength of the abdomen, hips, legs and feet reflect our physical vitality and centredness, and the strength of our connection with the ground. If the lower body is weak while the upper body is strong, a person may be relatively ungrounded and underconfident in dealing with physical or practical aspects of their lives. However, they may be quite mentally and socially active. The Intestine and Kidney Energies are frequently weak. Spending longer giving Shiatsu to the lower back, buttocks, lower abdomen, legs and feet can help bring the person's energy down to increase their vitality and groundedness. More Yin, expansive foods like sugar, fruits, spices, coffee and chocolate bring Energy upwards in the body. Reducing these foods and eating more grains, vegetables, beans and fish will help to bring the Energy down and strengthen the Energy in the lower body. More physical exercise using the legs, such as brisk walking, jogging or cycling can also help to bring Energy downwards to strengthen the lower body.

When the lower body appears stronger than the upper body, a person often enjoys being physically active, but can be 'overly grounded', without much reflection or thought about their lives. There may be a lot of stiffness and tension in the hips, legs, knees and ankles and excessive weight around the hips and thighs. If this condition has been present a long time, a person may develop osteoarthritis in the lower spine and hips. Shiatsu on the legs, and especially stretches in this part of the body, can help release this Energy so that it can move upwards to the upper body. Eating less of the more Yang, contractive foods like eggs, salt, meat and poultry and more of the balanced group of foods will also help reduce the excess of Energy in the lower body.

◆ The Head and Neck

A common problem in modern society, present in almost everyone, is tension in the neck and back of the head, sometimes resulting in headaches or migraines. One cause of this is probably the excessive amount of time we spend in intellectual thinking. Energy moves to whichever part of the body we are using, so if we use our 'heads' much of the time, this brings a lot of Energy up into the shoulders, neck and head. Another cause relates to the Liver and Gall Bladder, as the Meridians associated with these organs run over the back of the neck. People who eat or who have eaten a lot of meat, eggs and dairy foods, which greatly tax the Liver and Gall Bladder, generally have a lot of stiffness and tension in the back of the neck.

When the back of the neck becomes chronically tense, Energy can no longer move freely between the head and the body. Physically this can lead to headaches and problems with the eyes, ears and face. It can also trap people 'in their heads', so that they predominantly think, without their thoughts being connected to their feelings and actions, which require a flow of Energy between the head and the chest and abdomen. Also the person's thinking will tend to be rather intellectual and rigid. Shiatsu to the neck and head can release this tension, and often clears thoughts that have been persistently buzzing around a person's head, and help to reconnect them with their feelings. If the person is regularly eating meat, eggs and cheese, a reduction in these foods will also be of help.

When the head droops forwards, a person often has a dejected, depressed or defeated appearance. Their self-esteem and confidence may be low. Frequently the lower back is also weak, and the spine has a marked S shape. One cause of this inner collapse is weakness of the Energy in the Lungs and Large Intestine. People with this appearance commonly have problems in these organs, such as asthma, bronchitis, constipation, diarrhoea and intestinal cramps. The Lungs and Large Intestine are especially weakened by an excess of sweet foods, such as sugar, sweets, cakes, chocolate, honey, fruit and fruit juices. There may also be past experiences which have led to feeling dejected and a lack of belief in themselves. The chest and abdomen are generally Kyo, and more Shiatsu to these areas can help people with this drooping head posture. The balanced diet outlined in the last chapter will help to strengthen the Lungs and Large Intestine, and regular physical exercise which requires deep breathing can help in Energising these organs and the whole body.

◆ The Shoulders

The shoulders also reflect the health of the Lungs and Large Intestine. The two Meridians associated with these Organs run across the top of the shoulders. Emotionally, the shoulders relate to the shouldering of responsibilities, to work and action in the world. When the shoulders are raised, giving a defensive and fearful expression, the Lung and Large Intestine Meridians are usually weak or Kyo. Shiatsu on the front, top and back of the shoulders as well as down the arms will help to strengthen the Lung and Large Intestine Energy. The likely dietary cause of weakness of the Lungs and Large Intestine are described above in 'The Head and Neck'.

In many people the shoulders are pulled forwards, curving around the upper chest as if to protect it. There is often a feeling of being weighed down by too many responsibilities or psychological burdens. Such a person is prone to feeling depressed and withdrawn, preferring to spend much of their time alone and shunning company. Again the Lungs and Large Intestine are functioning poorly, and if the whole chest is sunken the heart and circulation may also be weak. The Lungs, Large Intestine and Heart may be too Yin or Yang, so eating the Energetically balanced diet is recommended. Breathing is often poor, so the body and brain are probably not receiving the full amount of oxygen they need. This may contribute to the mental depression and lack of Ki in the person. It is therefore very helpful to regularly take strong exercise where one has to breathe deeply. This often very quickly lifts the heavy or depressed feelings. Spending too much time alone should also be avoided. Sharing thoughts and feelings and having fun with other people can help in lifting the spirit and in opening the chest and shoulders.

◆ The Back

Backs are fascinating as they reflect the condition of all the organs of the body and the five Chakras or Energy centres governing our physical, emotional and mental disposition. Back pain is a very common problem. However, pains in the back are often considered to be a problem just of the back – the spine and the muscles and ligaments holding it in place. When considered Energetically, the back is a reflection of the inner health of the organs, and of their associated Meridians.

In the physical view the causes of back pain are generally a mystery, and only symptomatic treatment is offered. With an Energetic understanding the underlying causes of pains can usually be found, and steps taken to remedy them. With all pains, there is either an excess or deficiency of Ki in the area. By rebalancing the Ki with Shiatsu, the pain usually disappears. If the pain is long-standing or severe, changes in diet to improve the health of the organs associated with the particular area of the back may also be needed.

If there has been an imbalance in the Ki over a long period of time, the alignment of the vertebrae may also be out. Adjustments to return vertebrae to their proper position may remedy this. However, some people find that the vertebrae move out of place again. This is not surprising if there is still an Energetic imbalance. In these cases it can be helpful to rebalance the Energy in the area of misalignment with Shiatsu and possibly also make dietary changes. Once the Ki is balanced, the body itself will naturally tend to bring the spine into correct alignment. Adjustments will then be more successful. To understand the causes of back pain and postural imbalances we can divide the back into four areas.

The upper area is influenced by the Lungs and Heart, and so reflects a person's respiratory and circulatory functions. These organs are associated with our emotional expression and social nature. If this area appears weak or hollow or feels Kyo (soft, lacking in resistance) these organs and their associated Meridians are weak. The weakness may also be reflected in a weak-looking chest and drooping shoulders. The person may lack confident self-expression, and their circulation may be weak. Extra time giving Shiatsu to this area will help raise the Ki in these organs. More time on the chest and shoulders will probably be needed as well.

Sometimes the back is curved in this area, indicating that there has been a strong imbalance in Ki over a long period of time, and that the health of the Lungs and Heart is poorer. If the curve is great, there is a strong possibility that the person has experienced heart problems already. Shiatsu, and especially dietary changes are needed. The organs may be either overly Yin or Yang, so a balanced diet is recommended.

The second back area reflects the organs in the centre of the body: the Liver, Gall Bladder, Stomach, Pancreas, Spleen and Kidneys. Frequently there is a lot of tension in this part of the back, reflecting a build up of Energy in this central part of the torso. There may also be problems in these organs. This area of the back also reflects the activity of the solar plexus Chakra, which is concerned with our personal power and desires, and is the seat of our emotions. If there is much tension in this part of the back a person may be holding back in expressing or asserting themselves. They may be experiencing a lot of frustration, suppressed anger, or other strong emotions. Shiatsu to this area of the back and to the upper half of the abdomen can help dissipate this Energy. Often this tension is also associated with a diet high in animal foods, which cause an accumulation of Ki in these organs. Reducing these foods and eating a more Energetically balanced diet could then be of help.

The lower back is a common site of pain. It reflects the health of the Small and Large Intestines, which lie in front of this area, and of the Kidneys. The lower back is weak in the majority of people, because of poor health of the Intestines and Kidneys. It usually then feels soft, lacking in resilience. When the muscles around the spine are weak, lumbar vertebrae may also become misaligned in this area or, more severely, a person may experience a 'slipped disc'. So the original cause of slipped disc is usually poor health of the Intestines and Kidneys, due to an imbalanced diet and lifestyle! The base of the spine also represents our base – our physical vitality, sexual energy, and psychological groundedness. When this area is weak a person often experiences a lack of a strong root or base in their life.

During your Shiatsu, time spent holding any weak points or places which a person finds sensitive will help to strengthen the Ki in the lower back, and frequently is enough to get rid of back pain in this area. A severe weakness in this area is generally caused by the consumption of much of the more Yin foods. Eating the balanced diet, taking care not to consume too much fruit, fruit juices, stimulants, alcohol and other more Yin foods can be of great help to bring a long-term and permanent strengthening of the lower back and relief from any back pain in this area.

The sacrum and buttocks reflect the health of the bladder, the reproductive system and sexual organs. For example, during pregnancy, when the growing foetus puts pressure on the uterus, a woman frequently experiences pain over the sacrum. Shiatsu to the area is quite safe and can be of great help in relieving this pain. If this area appears strong, with well-rounded and firm buttocks, a person's overall vitality and sexual energy is probably strong. However, if there is tension in this area there may be excessive sexual desire, and a woman may suffer menstrual cramps. Shiatsu to disperse the Energy from the sacrum and buttocks can help diminish the cramps. Omitting animal foods like meat, eggs and poultry and excess salt will also be of benefit.

If the sacrum and buttocks are weak, with a lack of muscle tension in the buttocks, the bladder and reproductive functions are probably weak. In women there may well be an erratic menstrual cycle. In giving Shiatsu, spend longer holding points over the sacrum, and work deeply into the buttocks with your palms and thumbs. This can draw more Energy into this area and strengthen the associated organs. Considering diet, weakness in the lower body is usually caused by consuming an excess of Yin foods, especially sugar. Avoiding sugar and eating a balanced diet can help strengthen this area and a person's vitality and groundedness.

◆ The Legs

The legs and feet connect us with the ground. Energy passes from the ground into the soles of the feet and up the legs to the base and sacral Chakras and Hara. The strength of Ki in the legs reflects the strength of a person's Hara, and especially of the Intestines, Kidneys, and Reproductive Organs. If the Ki of the Hara and legs is strong, a person is likely to be in touch with the practical aspects of their life, and able to 'stand up for themselves'. However, if the Ki is weak here, the person may have difficulty dealing with the practical aspects of their lives, find it difficult to decide on their direction in life, and 'stand on their own feet'. They may trip up often, being unsure of their footing, both physically and in their life. When the legs are weak a person may subconsciously stiffen or brace their legs, tensing the muscles and locking the knee joints, so that they have a stiff-legged way of walking. Extra Shiatsu on the lower back, abdomen, legs and feet will help to strengthen the Ki in the legs. Such a person would also benefit from regular exercise with the legs, such as walking, jogging, cycling, or sports using the legs like football. This will draw Ki into the Hara and legs and strengthen them. Eating a lot of Yin foods has often contributed to this weakness, so a balanced diet with little or no sugar, spices, tea and coffee and tropical fruits will allow this area to become stronger.

The thighs reflect the strength of a person's sexual energy, especially the inside of the thigh. If this area is weak a person may develop knock knees. Extra Shiatsu here will strengthen the legs and Reproductive Organs. Exercise using the legs and a balanced diet will help to strengthen the thighs, as described above.

The knees are particularly affected by the condition of the middle organs of the body, the Liver, Gall Bladder, Stomach, Pancreas, Spleen and Kidneys. If there are pains, weakness or stiffness in the knees there is almost certainly an imbalance in these organs, which will also be reflected in the middle of the back and upper half of the abdomen. Pain in the front of the knees around the knee caps relates to the Stomach, Spleen and Pancreas. Pain on the inside and outside of the knees relates more to the Liver and Gall Bladder, and pain at the back of the knee relates to the Kidneys. Pain in the knees can be helped by using Kyo and Jitsu. If the area of pain feels weak, soft and empty, it needs to be tonified by holding the sensitive points. If the area is tense and full, it needs to be relaxed by moving the Energy away from the area. If you are not sure which to do, give a moderate amount of Shiatsu on the painful area and above and below on the thigh and lower leg. There are a variety of dietary causes of knee pains, which are too detailed to explain here. A balanced diet will help most cases and can be recommended.

The calves reflect the health of the Intestines, Bladder and Kidneys. If the calf muscles are painful when touched, or swollen or hard, it indicates that the Intestines are not in a good condition. Shiatsu on the calves will help to get the Energy flowing in the

Intestines, and relax the calves as well. Reducing the more extreme Yin and Yang foods and eating more of the Energetically balanced foods will improve the health of the Intestines and so improve the condition of the calves.

If a person frequently gets cramps in the calves and/or in the soles of the feet, there is an imbalance in the Kidney and Bladder Meridians. Shiatsu down the back and backs of the legs and on the soles of the feet often helps to remedy this problem. Cutting down on more extreme foods that have a detrimental affect on the health of the Kidneys, especially excess salt and drinks like tea, coffee, alcohol and tropical fruit juices, will also improve Kidney functioning and therefore help reduce the cramping.

The ankles are related to the Kidneys and Reproductive Organs. Puffiness or swelling around the ankles is generally caused by the Kidneys functioning poorly, so that excess fluid is not efficiently removed from the body. Shiatsu down the whole of the back of the body and around the ankles and on the soles of the feet can help, along with the dietary changes already mentioned above.

If there is weakness in the ankles a person is prone to twisting their ankles, and they may find them very sensitive when you give Shiatsu to them. However, more Shiatsu is needed to strengthen the Energy in the ankles, though not enough to cause too much pain.

◆ The Feet

The feet can tell us an amazing amount through Oriental diagnosis. The health of all the major organs in the body is reflected in the feet. The shape of the feet also particularly reflects the quality of our contact with the ground and with the practical realities in our life.

We use our feet to step forward in life. If the feet appear strong with a well curved arch, a person's Intestines and Kidneys are probably functioning well, and they probably have a strong will and self-determination. They are likely to do a lot in life. If the feet appear rather lifeless, maybe with a weak arch making the foot look flat, there may be weakness in the Kidneys and Intestines, and the person will tend to lack a firm footing in their life. An excess of more Yin foods is often one cause of this weakness. Firm Shiatsu to the ankles, soles, and toes will help to Energize the feet and the whole body.

Sometimes the toes appear to be clasping the ground, and there is a lot of tension in the upper side of the feet. Usually the Liver and Gall Bladder Meridians that run from the first and fourth toes up the top of the foot are Jitsu, causing tension that pulls the toes into their clasping position. Generally the Liver and Gall Bladder have become too Yang from the consumption of a lot of meat, eggs, poultry and salt, so a reduction in these foods and a more balanced diet will improve the health of these organs and help the feet straighten. Shiatsu with the thumb along the grooves between the metatarsal bones on the upper side of the feet will help shift the excess Ki that has built up here, helping the toes straighten and enhancing the functioning of the Liver and Gall Bladder. When the toes curl in this way, a person frequently has a rather rigid outlook on life, and resists changes. They may be happier if they can try to become more flexible and open-minded, and accept change and new ideas in their lives.

When some people lie on their back, their feet droop downwards away from the head, due to the upper side of the feet being Kyo. This indicates that the chest, Lungs and Heart are also Kyo. The person's personal spirit or sense of themselves may be low. Shiatsu

135

to the feet and chest will be beneficial. Usually they have consumed a lot of Yin foods, and often lack regular physical exercise. A balanced diet with little of the extreme Yin foods will help to strengthen the chest. Encouragement to express inner feelings and desires may also be appropriate.

◆ The Abdomen

Like the back, the abdomen reflects the health of the whole person. The quality of Energy in the twelve Meridians can be diagnosed in the abdomen by a skilled Shiatsu practitioner. At this stage in learning Shiatsu we are going to look more generally at the abdomen and what you can easily diagnose now.

The lower half of the abdomen from the navel downwards reflects the strength of the Hara, the centre of Energy and vitality for the whole body and being. The Energetic condition is generally the same as the area directly behind it, the lower back, so if during your Shiatsu you found the lower back to be weak, then the Hara will probably also be weak. Ideally this centre is full of Ki, which creates a slight bulge in the lower abdomen (not the whole abdomen!) with a bouncy, resilient but not hard and tense feel to the area. Such a person will probably have a lot of physical and mental energy, a healthy sexual drive, and a strong centredness and confidence. If the lower abdomen is weak, you will find that you can push into it easily with little resistance. The person may be feeling fatigued or stressed. Pushing in and holding in the lower abdomen will help draw Ki into the Hara, and also strengthen the Kidneys and Intestines. A weak Hara is often created by eating a lot of Yin foods like sugar, fruits, tea and coffee. A balanced diet with plenty of whole grains, vegetables, sea vegetables and soups seasoned with miso will help to strengthen the Hara. Physical exercise using the legs can also be helpful.

When you are giving Shiatsu to the centre of the abdomen around the navel, pushing in deeply with your fingers you will feel the Small Intestine. Often on pushing in your fingers will hit what feels like a rock inside. This is tension in the Intestine. The Intestine is mostly muscle, and like any muscle on the outside of the body, it can become chronically tense and hard. Obviously when the intestine is cramped like this, digestion cannot be so efficient, and the Energy being held here would be more useful circulating around the whole body. Tension in the Intestines can be caused by withholding emotions, and also by a poor diet. Gentle holding on this tense area will often result in it relaxing, releasing a lot of Energy and inner tension.

The upper half of the abdomen above the navel contains the middle organs: the Liver, Gall Bladder, Stomach, Spleen and Pancreas. This area should be flexible, so that your fingers can sink deeply into the area and under the ribs. Unfortunately this is often not the case, the area is more often hard due to a build up and stagnation of Energy in this part of the body. A typical modern diet containing animal foods, sugar and refined foods creates a stagnation of Energy in these organs. This area also reflects the solar plexus Chakra, the centre of personal power. Repressing one's feelings and emotions over a long period of time creates a build up of tension in this area and in the diaphragm, the sheet of muscle that separates the chest cavity containing the Lungs and Heart from the abdominal cavity containing the Stomach, Intestines, Kidneys, Pancreas and Spleen, Liver and Gall Bladder. Shiatsu in the upper abdomen and over the lower ribs when giving Shiatsu to the chest helps release this tension. You may have to be patient in slowly getting the accumulated Ki to move out of the area.

Some people find it almost unbearable to have their abdomen touched by another person at all. They might feel threatened and vulnerable even by the thought of being touched here. These people generally have a great deal of unresolved emotional tension held in the abdomen, and their fear is actually of releasing these emotions so that they have to experience them and face up to them. It is obviously desirable that they should do this, but great sensitivity and compassion will be needed. Be prepared for them bursting into tears!

◆ The Chest

The chest reflects the health of the Heart and the circulation, and also the Heart Chakra which is the centre of love, compassion, and feeling. In Chinese teachings the Heart is the store place of Shen, our individual spirit that guides us through life. When it is active we feel happy and alive, when it is relatively inactive we feel sad and dead. The Heart of small children is usually 'open', and they feel a lot, and are alive and spirited, as well as being vulnerable. During our life we frequently 'close' our heart to protect it against being hurt. But as it closes, so does our ability to feel, to live, and be alive in following our Hearts.

Often the chest looks collapsed or hollow, and the person may look resigned and in need of support. Their circulation is generally weak, giving a pale complexion. The chest then needs to be treated sensitively, rough Shiatsu could cause the Heart to close further. Gentle but firm Shiatsu, with more holding to bring Ki into this area, can help the chest and Heart open. The person may like to share some of the feelings that have caused their Hearts to close. Exercise involving deep breathing can also help by bringing more Ki into the chest.

Sometimes the chest appears over-inflated and expanded, and is Jitsu. The circulation is often over-active, possibly resulting in high blood pressure. Such a person can seem confident and assertive, but underneath they may be frightened of letting go. Shiatsu can help move the excess Energy out of the area, and loosen the muscles so that the chest relaxes.

◆ The Arms

As a whole the arms and hands are primarily fed by Energy from the Heart and throat Chakras, so the strength of Ki in the arms is closely connected with what is happening in the chest. For example, when the chest is Kyo, the arms and hands are usually weak also. The arms and hands could be called 'the wings of the Heart', they are used for giving and receiving, and are used much in expressing our feelings. When giving Shiatsu to the arms it can be useful to consider them along with the chest – if the chest, arms and hands are Kyo as a whole then they all need to be tonified; if they are all Jitsu then they all need to be sedated.

The inside of the upper arm is especially connected with the Heart as the Heart Meridian passes along here. (Interestingly, this is where pain is usually felt during a heart attack.) If this area seems particularly weak and flabby, the Heart Meridian is low in Energy, and extra Shiatsu to this area will be beneficial.

The elbows, like the knees, are associated with the middle organs of the body: the Liver, Gall Bladder, Stomach, Spleen and Pancreas. Pains or other problems around the elbows are usually associated with an Energy imbalance in the middle organs, which can also be diagnosed in the middle back, upper abdomen, knees and feet. If there are pains in the elbows, such as in tennis elbow, you can give Shiatsu to the painful places, if possible diagnosing whether they are Kyo or Jitsu and treating them appropriately. The dietary causes of the pain could be various, so recommendations apart from eating the balanced diet cannot be given here.

The wrists, like the ankles, are energetically connected with the Kidneys and Reproductive Organs. A person's wrists may look weak, making them prone to spraining or breaking them. The skin may also be darker around the wrist than on the rest of the arm, especially on the inside of the arm. This indicates poor health in the Kidneys and Reproductive Organs. When the wrists are weak, extra time can be spent giving Shiatsu to them, especially pressing with the thumb into the groove between the bones of the lower arm and those of the hand.

◆ The Hands

The hands as a whole are closely connected to the Heart and circulation, although like the feet they also reflect the health condition of all the organs of the body. If the hands overall appear weak and rather lifeless, the person's Heart Energy and circulation is probably also weak. They may have difficulties with their emotional expression, with giving and receiving. Firm Shiatsu to the palms and fingers can help Energize the hands, warm the Heart, and improve circulation.

On the other hands the hands may be very warm, possibly red and swollen, and tense. The Heart and circulation is probably over-active, and the person tense overall. With an over-active Heart there may also be a tendency to high blood pressure. Shiatsu over the hands and fingers can draw some of this excess Energy off, relieving the tension and helping a person feel calmer and more relaxed.

This chapter has given you a lot of information, which hopefully will provide a basis for your continued experimentation with giving Shiatsu. As you progress to perceiving and working with imbalances in different areas of the body, don't lose sight of the overall needs of a person. There is a danger in becoming preoccupied with giving Shiatsu to detailed areas and losing touch with the needs of an individual as a whole. You may then be effective in working on particular areas, but the overall effect on a person may not be so good. So try to keep in mind the overall needs of your friend while you are giving Shiatsu over their body.

Chapter 11

INCORPORATING TSUBOS INTO YOUR SHIATSU

In this chapter, a number of the Tsubos or acupuncture points most commonly used in acupuncture, acupressure and Shiatsu are listed, with their numbers, names in English, and precise location and common uses. Particular points have specific effects due to a number of Energetic relationships with the rest of the body.

1. A Tsubo frequently has an effect on the Energy in its local area of the body. For example, a number of points around the shoulder are useful for relieving pain and other problems in the shoulder.

2. Giving Shiatsu to a Tsubo affects the Energy flow along the Meridian that it lies on. A Tsubo may then be useful for a problem that is associated with an imbalance of Energy in another part of its Meridian. For example, Large Intestine 4 in the hand can be used to help alleviate toothache as this Meridian runs from the hand to the face.

3. Tsubos can be used to create changes in the internal Organs of the body, via the Meridians they lie on. So Lung 1 on the inside of the shoulder can benefit Lung problems like asthma and coughing, and Large Intestine 4 can help constipation and other Large Intestine problems.

4. There are a number of other relationships between specific Tsubos and the rest of the body, based on more complex Oriental theories than this introductory book can cover. Some of the books given in the Further Reading section can be consulted for this information.

You can use this list in two ways. Firstly, if you or somebody you are going to give Shiatsu to has a particular health problem, consult the list and find any points that are indicated as being commonly useful for that problem. Look at the locations of the Tsubos on the charts and read the description of their locations, and then find them either on your own or on the receiver's body. From the chart and description you should be able to get quite close to the actual Tsubo on the body, but to find it precisely you now need to 'feel about' until you feel you are right on it. Very often when you precisely find a Tsubo, your thumb or finger 'falls' into a little depression, and the point feels more sensitive than the surrounding area when pressed. You may also just intuitively feel, 'I've got it!'

When giving Shiatsu to another person, these Tsubos are ideally incorporated into their full-body treatment. Give Shiatsu to the Tsubos as you come to them in your full-body treatment, rather than working on them separately. If you do not have the time to give a full treatment, you could just apply pressure to the points, but the receiver will get much more benefit if you also give them a full-body treatment. If you are using Tsubos on yourself, you will unfortunately only be able to use the points!

The second way of using this list is that while giving Shiatsu you will discover points that feel as if they particularly need holding. These points are often, but by no means always,

recognized acupuncture points. You can consult the list to see if
the points you have discovered are recognized accupunture points,
and if so, their names, numbers and common uses. In this way
you can learn from the body of knowledge built up from other
people's experience.

I would recommend using this list in both of these ways.
Over-dependence on the first method can stunt the development of
your own sensitivity and trust in what you discover through
touching the body. As your sense of touch develops, you will
actually find the points on a particular person's body that are most
in need of Shiatsu, and that will give the greatest benefits. Trust what
you feel through your touch more than what you read in a book!

When you use specific Tsubos, use the points on both sides of the
body. The points can be held anything from half a minute to two
minutes. Apply pressure while observing the Basic Principles for
Giving Shiatsu described in Chapter 5. In particular, make sure that
your pressure is exactly at right-angles to the body surface at the
point. Then your Ki penetrates to the bottom of the Tsubo and has
the maximum beneficial effect. Even if the angle is only slightly out,
you will not reach the bottom, and the effect is greatly reduced.

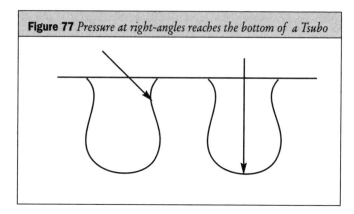

Figure 77 *Pressure at right-angles reaches the bottom of a Tsubo*

When you press a Tsubo you may well feel that the Energy at the point is full, with greater muscle tone, or more Jitsu. You then need to press the point in such a way as to disperse the excess Energy. Simple holding may be enough, or you may find that making small circular movements with your thumb or 'pumping' your thumb in and out more effective, until you feel the excess Energy subside and the excess muscle tone relax. On the other hand, Energy at the point may be lacking, so that the Tsubo feels deficient, 'needy', and unusually soft. Energy needs to be brought into such Kyo points, by simply holding them for some time. As you hold you may well be able to feel the point 'filling up' with Energy, and the muscle tone increase slightly. For more detailed information on the diagnosis and treatment of Kyo and Jitsu, refer back to Chapter 8.

There are some points that should not be used during pregnancy, as they give strong stimulation to the uterus and could cause a miscarriage. These are clearly marked in the list, so please avoid them if there is any possibility of your receiver being pregnant.

In describing the location of Tsubos the Oriental term 'cun' is used. 1 cun is the width of the receiver's thumb at the widest point. The width of the first and second fingers is approximately 1^1/2 cun, and the width of the 4 fingers is approximately 3 cun. If your hands are about the same size as the receiver's, then you can use your own fingers to make these measurements.

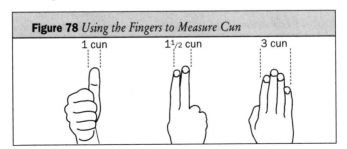

Figure 78 *Using the Fingers to Measure Cun*

Figure 79a *Charts for Finding the Tsubo*

LG Lung
LI Large Intestine
ST Stomach
SP Spleen
HT Heart
SI Small Intestine
BL Bladder
KD Kidney
HG Heart Governor
TH Triple Heater
GB Gall Bladder
LV Liver
GV Governing Vessel
CV Conception Vessel

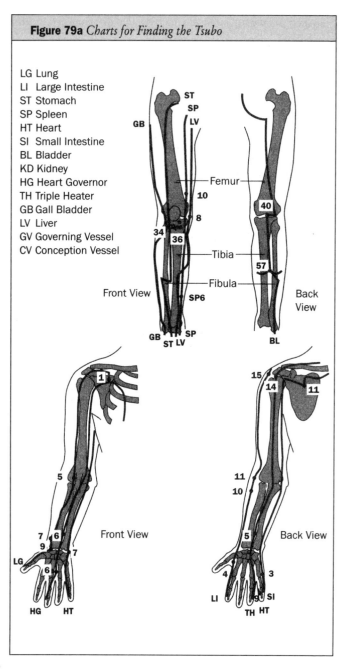

ST
SP
GB
LV
Femur
10
8
34
36
Tibia
Fibula
Front View
SP6
GB SP
ST LV

Back
View
Femur
40
Tibia
57
BL

1
5
7 6
9
7
LG
6
HG   HT
Front View

15
14   11
11
10
5
4   3
LI
9 SI
TH HT
Back View

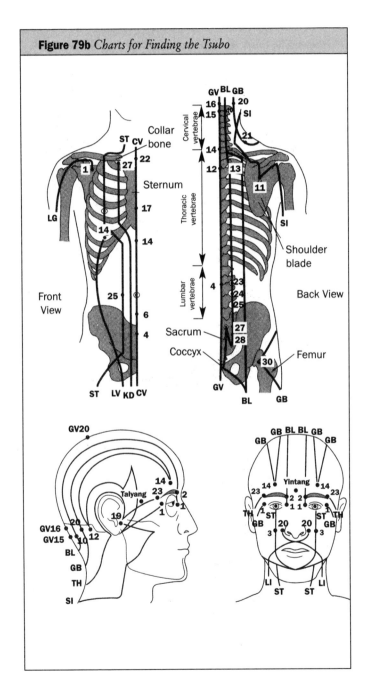

Figure 79b *Charts for Finding the Tsubo*

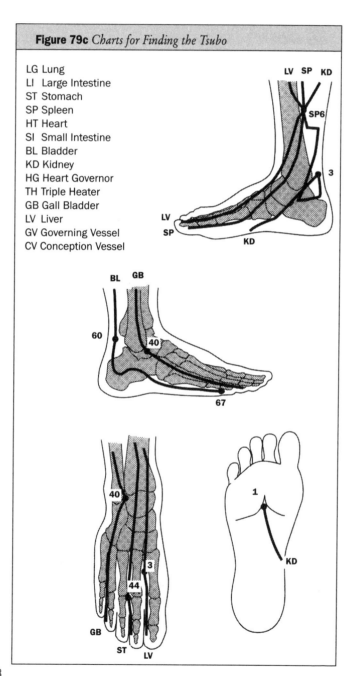

Figure 79c *Charts for Finding the Tsubo*

LG Lung
LI Large Intestine
ST Stomach
SP Spleen
HT Heart
SI Small Intestine
BL Bladder
KD Kidney
HG Heart Governor
TH Triple Heater
GB Gall Bladder
LV Liver
GV Governing Vessel
CV Conception Vessel

Number Name in English	Location	Common Uses
LUNG		
1 Centre of Gathering	Between 1st and 2nd ribs, 1 cun below middle of collar bone.	Asthma, coughs, common cold, breathing difficulties, pain in chest, shoulder pain.
5 In the Groove	On end of elbow crease on thumb side of arm.	Elbow pain and swelling, tonsillitis, painful breathing, coughs, asthma, fever associated with lung problems.
7 Broken Sequence	1¹/2 cun above wrist crease on thumb side of arm.	Congestion, headaches, colds, coughing, Bell's palsy, stiff neck.
9 Great Stagnation	On wrist crease in indentation below thumb.	Reviving unconscious person, coughs, painful breathing, pharyngitis, pain and paralysis of wrist.
LARGE INTESTINE		
4 Great Eliminator	On tip of fleshy mound which is formed by drawing thumb into index finger.	Normalizes intestines, general well-being, facial problems e.g. frontal headache, neuralgia, lower toothache, problems of back of hand. DON'T USE DURING PREGNANCY.
10 Arm Three Miles	1¹/2 cun below the end of the crease formed by bending elbow.	Sore throat, general well-being, pain or fatigue in arms.
11 Lake of Energy on the Corner	End of crease formed by bending elbow.	Hypertension, tennis elbow, haemorrhoids.
15 Corner of the Shoulder	In indentation on outside of shoulder bone.	Frozen shoulder, neuralgia of arm and shoulder, hemiplegia.
20 Welcome Fragrance	In groove at wide point of nostrils.	Sinusitis, facial tension, neuralgia of face, paralysis of facial nerves.

Number Name in English	Location	Common Uses
STOMACH		
3 Empty Space in Bone	Directly below pupil in space under cheekbone.	Sinus and nasal congestion, facial tension or paralysis, upper toothache, neuralgia of face.
25 Heavenly Pivot	2 cun either side of the navel.	Abdominal pain, menstrual pain, bowel irregularities, intestinal obstruction.
36 Leg Three Miles	In depression outside the tibia 3 cun below the kneecap.	Well-being particularly for tonifying Stomach and Spleen Meridians, fatigue, tired legs, loss of appetite.
44 Inner Garden	Between 2nd & 3rd toe division, pushing in towards 2nd toe.	Stomach pain, toothache, frontal headache, sore throat.
SPLEEN		
6 Meeting Point of the Three Yin Leg Meridians	3 cun above the tip of ankle bone, push in to the edge of the tibia.	Ankle pains, menstrual pain, digestive problems, female reproductive problems, insomnia, overweight. **DON'T USE DURING PREGNANCY.**
10 Ocean of Blood	3 cun above the kneecap on bulge of muscle.	Itching, hives, menstrual pain.
HEART		
7 Gate of God	On wrist crease in indentation below little finger.	Reviving unconscious person, insomnia, hysteria, high blood pressure, irritability, angina pectoris.
9 Little Rushing In	Inside the little finger about 0.1 cun from the corner of the nail.	Heart attack, severe anxiety, hysteria, angina pectoris.

Number Name in English	Location	Common Uses
SMALL INTESTINE		
3 Back Stream	On crease formed by making a fist on edge of hand below little finger.	Paralysis of fingers, numbness, hardness of hearing, ringing in ears.
11 Centre of Heaven	Two thirds up mid-line of shoulder blade.	Shoulder pain, frozen shoulder, intercostal neuralgia, lung problems.
19 Palace of Hearing	In the depression between the jaw joint and the middle part of the ear.	Ringing in ears, difficulty in hearing.
BLADDER		
1 Eye Brightness	Inner corner of eye.	Poor or tired vision, swollen eyes.
2 Collecting Bamboo	In notch directly above Bladder 1.	Front or back headache, hayfever, eye strain.
10 Pillar of Heaven	Below back of skull, 1 cun to the sides of the middle of the neck.	Headaches, insomnia, nasal congestion, neck ache, eye and nose problems.
13 Lung Back Transporting Point	1.5 cun to the sides of the spine, level with the space between the 3rd and 4th thoracic vertebrae.	Cough, asthma, breathlessness, bronchitis, pneumonia. Tonifies deficient Lungs.
23 Kidney Back Transporting Point	1.5 cun to the sides of the spine, level with the space between the 2nd and 3rd lumbar vertebrae.	Tonifies Kidneys, impotence, infertility, lack of sexual desire, physical weakness and exhaustion, depression, lack of will-power, chronic low back pain, weak legs, chronic ear problems e.g. tinnitus, deafness; poor vision.
24 Sea of Ki Back Transporting Point	1.5 cun to the sides of the space between the 3rd and 4th lumbar vertebrae.	Chronic or acute lower back pain, irregular menstruation, uterine bleeding.

Number Name in English	Location	Common Uses
25 Large Intestine Back Transporting Point	1.5 cun to the sides of the space between the 4th and 5th lumbar vertebrae.	Tonifies Large Intestine, constipation or diarrhoea, abdominal distension, chronic or acute lower back pain.
27 Small Intestine Back Transporting Point	At level of 1st depression in the sacrum, 1.5 cun out from the centre of the sacrum.	Any small intestine problem e.g. abdominal pain; back pain over sacrum, urination and menstruation problems.
28 Bladder Back Transporting Point	At level of 2nd depression in the sacrum, 1.5 cun out from the centre of the sacrum.	Bladder problems e.g. difficult urination, retention of urine, bed-wetting; strengthens lower back.
40 Supporting Middle	In middle of crease behind knee.	Lower back ache, calf spasms, sciatica.
57 In the Mountain	In depression in centre of calf muscle.	Sciatica, tired legs, calf spasms, pain on sole of foot.
60 Mountain	On the outside of the ankle between the ankle bone and Achilles tendon.	Sciatica, dizziness, backache. **DON'T USE DURING PREGNANCY.**
67 Extreme Yin	Outside of the little toe, at base of toenail.	Malposition of foetus, headaches, blurred vision, pain in eyes and other eye problems. **DON'T USE DURING PREGNANCY.**

KIDNEY

Number Name in English	Location	Common Uses
1 Bubbling Spring	In the crease in the middle of the ball of the foot.	General vitality, fear, dizziness, revival.
3 Greater Stream	Between tip of ankle bone and Achilles tendon.	General kidney function, pain in lower back, impotence, abnormal menstruation, deficient Kidney Energy.
27 Transportation Place	Between 1st rib and collar bone.	Bronchitis, chest pain, asthma.

Number Name in English	Location	Common Uses
HEART GOVERNOR		
6 Inside Gate	2 cun above wrist crease between tendons in the middle of the forearm.	Nausea, vomiting, sea sickness, insomnia, heart palpitations.
8 Palace of Anxiety	Cup hand, at bottom of the 'cup' in the palm.	Exhaustion, shyness, high blood pressure, writer's cramp.
TRIPLE HEATER		
5 Outer Gate	2 cun above wrist crease on back of arm.	Tinnitus, ear infection, migraine headaches, aversion to cold.
14 Top of Shoulder	Just behind the tip of the shoulder bone.	Shoulder joint pain.
23 Silk Bamboo Hollow	At outside tip of eyebrow in depression on bone around eye.	Headache, eye and ear problems.
GALL BLADDER		
1 Hole in Bone for Eye	Outside corner of eye in depression on bone around eye.	Headache around temples, conjunctivitis, eye problems.
12 Whole Bone	Depression below the back edge of the skull and behind the bone behind the ear.	Headache, toothache, ringing in ear.
14 Pure Yang	1 cun above the middle of the eyebrow.	Front headaches, sinus blockage, eye problems.
20 Windy Pond	Below the back edge of the skull, between the back and side neck muscles.	Eye disorders, common cold, front and side headaches, hypertension, tension in neck, dizziness, vertigo.

Number Name in English	Location	Common Uses
21 Shoulder Well	A little behind the highest point of the shoulder in line with the 7th cervical vertebra.	Shoulder pain, frozen shoulder, mastitis, lack of milk, childbirth difficulties. DON'T USE DURING PREGNANCY.
30 Jumping Circle	One-third of the way between the head of the femur and the coccyx in the side of the buttocks.	Sciatica, lumbar pain, lumbago, arthritis or rheumatism in hip area, hip problems.
34 Yang Hill Spring	In the depression behind and below the head of the fibula.	Ankle pains, headaches, knee problems, leg weakness.
40 Mound Ruins	In depression in front of and slightly below the ankle bone.	Lumbago, aids function of liver and gall bladder, neck pain, calf pain.

LIVER

3 Bigger Rushing	1.5 cun above bridge of 1st & 2nd toes.	Headaches, dizziness, muscle cramps and muscle tension.
8 Spring on the Corner	On inside of knee joint, above bent knee crease.	Inside knee problems, urine retention, burning urination, itchy genitals.
14 Gate of Hope	Between 6th & 7th ribs directly below nipple.	Rib pain, lactation problems, coughing, breathing difficulty.

GOVERNING VESSEL

4 Gate of Life	Between 2nd & 3rd lumbar vertebrae.	Strengthens Kidneys, lumbar weakness, lack of vitality, impotence, infertility, weak legs.
12 Body Pillar	Between 3rd & 4th thoracic vertebrae.	Asthma, colds, calms nervous system, strengthens whole body.
14 Big Vertebra	Between 7th cervical and 1st thoracic vertebrae.	Common cold, fever, asthma, headaches, clears mind and stimulates brain.

Number Name in English	Location	Common Uses
15 Gate of Fool	Between 1st and 2nd cervical vertebrae.	Colds, headaches, nosebleeds; stimulates speech, so good for speech difficulties.
16 Wind Palace	Between skull and 1st cervical vertebra.	Stimulates/calms brain, giddiness, tension in upper neck.
20 Hundred Meetings	At the centre of head on middle of line connecting tops of ears.	Headaches, giddiness, piles, prolapsed anus or vagina.

CONCEPTION VESSEL

4 Gate to Original Ki	3 cun below navel.	Strengthens overall Ki and body and mind, deficient Kidney Energy, fatigue, grounding, reproductive organ problems.
6 Ocean of Ki	1.5 cun below navel.	Physical and mental exhaustion and depression, lower abdominal pain or distension, lack of willpower.
14 Great Palace	1 cun below lower tip of breastbone.	Acts on stomach and heart, stomach spasm, stomach ulcers, emotional upset, calms mind.
17 Middle of Chest	On breastbone directly between nipples.	Acts on heart and lungs. Pain or fullness in chest, breathlessness, chronic cough or bronchitis, palpitations, high blood pressure, asthma, angina pectoris.
22 Heaven Projection	Between the inside ends of the collar bones.	Acute and chronic cough and asthma, bronchitis, sore throat.

Number Name in English	Location	Common Uses
EXTRA POINTS NOT LYING ON MERIDIANS		
Yintang Seal Hall	Between the eyebrows.	Calms mind and tension in forehead, frontal headaches, blocked frontal sinuses.
Taiyang Greater Yang	In depression 1 cun behind the middle of the outer end of the eyebrow and outer corner of the eye.	Headaches in the side of the head, over-active mind, eye problems.
Xiyan Knee Eyes	Two points in the depressions at the lower outside corners of the kneecap.	Pain in front of knee or deep inside joint.

Chapter 12

MERIDIAN EXERCISES FOR YOURSELF

T his chapter describes some stretching exercises that promote Energy flow in the twelve main Meridians, called Makko-ho exercises. They are widely taught along with Shiatsu as a way of improving health, and of assessing the condition of the Energy flow within one's own Meridians. They are quite simple, and take about ten minutes to run through. Ideally they can be practised daily, for example in the morning after getting up. They can also be used as a part of other exercise programmes, or at any time of the day when the body feels in need of some rejuvenation.

There are six exercises, each stretching one pair of Meridians. Stretching a Meridian has the effect of stimulating Energy to flow along that Meridian. By stretching all the Meridians with the six exercises, one's entire Energy flow through the Meridian System is improved. This often has the benefits of removing tiredness (which is often due to stuck Energy flow rather than a lack of Energy as often thought) and making the body feel lighter. Stretching the Meridians also has the effect of rebalancing the Energy flow in the Meridian system. If a Meridian is Jitsu, the stretch helps to move the excess Energy out of the Meridian. If it is Kyo, more Energy will be brought into the deficient Meridian.

In order to promote Energy flow, these exercises must be done in a particular way. Many other stretching exercises are performed to have a physical effect, and it is thought best to stretch as far as possible regardless of the tension and pain it may produce. The body may also be 'bounced' to stretch that little bit further. While this kind of stretching may increase physical flexibility, it has little effect on Energy flow, as pain and tension prevents the flow of Energy. (You will find that practising the Makko-ho exercises is actually a very effective way of increasing your flexibility, painlessly.)

The Makko-ho exercises are performed quite differently so as to have the maximum effect on Energy. Firstly, one stays relaxed throughout, with smooth, continuous breathing. One only moves into the stretch position as far as is needed to feel a stretch in the particular Meridian pair, without any force, so that you can stay relaxed. Secondly, the stretch is held for some time, from half a minute to several minutes, to give time for the Energy to move, rather than a quick 'in and out' motion. After holding a particular stretch for 5, 10 or 15 seconds, you may feel a moment in time when any stiffness or slight pain begins to recede, and the stretch becomes much easier. This is the moment when Ki begins to flow. Once Energy starts flowing you obviously want to hold the stretch longer so that as much Energy as possible is set moving. With a quick stretch or bouncing movement, this moment is never reached.

Besides the health benefits of the Makko-ho exercises, they can also be used to assess the relative condition of your six pairs of Meridians. If you feel a lot of stiffness and resistance with a restricted amount of movement in a particular stretch, it indicates that that pair of Meridians is more Jitsu. On the other hand if a stretch feels easier with a greater amount of movement, and feels particularly pleasurable, the Meridian pair being stretched is probably more Kyo. Some people who generally find stretching exercises very easy actually have a lot of Kyo Meridians. When you run through all six stretches, it will probably become clear which of your Meridian pairs are most out of balance. If you practise the Makko-ho exercises regularly you will be able to observe these most imbalanced Meridians gradually coming into balance. You may also like to choose to practise the stretches for your most imbalanced Meridians more often, to produce a quicker rebalancing and improvement in your health.

The Makko-ho exercises can also be used as a basis for other stretching-type exercises. Once you are familiar with the location of the Meridians, you can experiment with yoga asanas and other exercises to see which Meridians they most effectively stretch. You can then select other stretching exercises to work on particular Meridians.

◆ How to Perform the Exercises

1. Before you begin the exercises, make sure that you are relaxed and centred. You could practise Abdominal Breathing (as described in Chapter 5) for a few minutes before you begin.

2. Before each stretch, take a breath in, then breathe out as you go into the stretch. As you hold the stretch position, keep breathing evenly and continuously. Holding the breath holds tension in the body, whereas with continuous breathing tension is released on each out breath. Then, as you rise out of the stretch, take a deep breath in, then breathe out and relax.

3. Only move as far into each stretch position as you will be able to remain in for a while, without creating discomfort and tension throughout your body. You should be able to feel

a stretch along the pair of Meridians, but this should not be so much as to cause pain.

4. Hold the stretch for half a minute to several minutes. See if you can feel the moment at which Energy begins to move, and the position begins to feel more comfortable. As more Energy flows you may well find that you can move a little further into the stretch.

5. After completing all six exercises, a lot of Energy will have been set moving. If you immediately jump up and start rushing about, you will stop this movement. So, rather like after receiving a Shiatsu treatment, it is a good idea to lie down for a few minutes to allow the Energy to keep flowing and come to a new balance. When you feel ready, get up, and try to keep the feeling of being relaxed and centred as you go about your day's activities.

◆ Lung and Large Intestine Meridian Stretch

Stand with your feet shoulder width apart, hook your thumbs together behind your back and stretch your fingers outwards. As you breathe out, bend forwards, keeping the legs and arms straight. Bring your hands as far over the head as possible without using force – imagine that somebody else is pulling your hands forward. The feeling should be of an enjoyable stretch. Check your body to make sure that you are not tensing up, and breathe slowly as you hold the position for half a minute or more. You may well be able to feel a particularly strong stretch along the Lung and Large Intestine Meridians in the shoulders, arms and thumbs. Finally, breathe in as you slowly straighten up to a standing position.

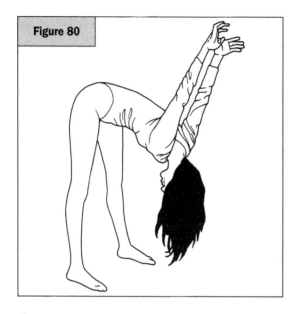

Figure 80

◆ Spleen and Stomach Meridian Stretch

Kneel on the floor, and move your feet outwards so that your bottom sits on the floor. If your bottom does not reach the floor, put a cushion under it so that your body weight is resting through your bottom on the floor. Now, as you breathe out, lean backwards and support your weight on your hands behind you. You may now feel a stretch along the Spleen and Stomach Meridians on the front of your thighs and calves. If it feels that you are getting plenty of stretch in this position and that you could not comfortably stretch any further, stay in this position for at least half a minute, breathing evenly.

If you feel that you need to stretch further, drop down onto your elbows. Make sure your knees are within a few inches of each other and on the floor – if they splay outwards or upwards the Meridians are not so effectively stretched. Again, if this is as far as you can comfortably go, stay in this position; don't think that you have to force yourself further. It is so important to be able to stay relaxed while stretching. If, however, you feel that you could quite easily stretch further, drop your back onto the floor. Raise your arms over your head and interlock the fingers to increase the stretching of these Meridians in the abdomen and chest. If you feel discomfort or pain in your lower back, don't force yourself to stay in this position, go back to resting on your elbows. After half a minute or so raise yourself back onto your elbows, then onto your hands, then sit up straight.

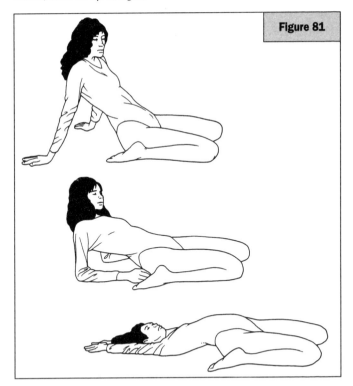

Figure 81

◆ Heart and Small Intestine Meridian Stretch

Sit on the floor and draw the soles of your feet together. Grasp your feet with your hands and pull the feet as close to the body as possible. Make sure your elbows are outside your legs, and as you breathe out lean forward, taking your head towards or onto your feet. Hold this position for at least half a minute, breathing evenly. This is not such a strenuous stretch as the last two, but you will probably be able to feel a line of tension along the Heart and Small Intestine Meridians on the underside of the arms. Finally, breathe in as you rise out of the stretch position, and relax.

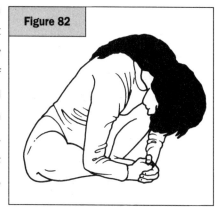

Figure 82

◆ Kidney and Bladder Meridian Stretch

Sit on the floor with your legs straight out in front of you and bend forwards from the hips, reaching with your hands as far down the legs as you can comfortably go. You may be able to hold onto your feet or, if you cannot stretch that far, your ankles. Drop your head forwards to stretch the Bladder Meridian in the back of the neck. You should now be able to feel a line of stretch in the Kidney and Bladder

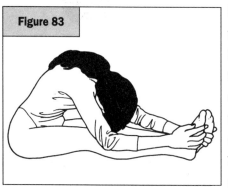

Figure 83

Meridians all the way from your feet, up the backs of the legs, in the back and neck. Hold the position for half a minute or more, as usual, making sure that your breathing is free and easy and your body is relaxed. Then rise back up to a sitting position as you breathe in.

◆ Heart Governor and Triple Heater Meridian Stretch

Sit on the floor either with the soles of your feet together or with the feet crossed over each other, whichever is more comfortable. Now cross your arms over each other and grasp your knees with your hands wrapped well around the knees. Take a breath in, and then as you breathe out drop your head and body forwards and your knees downwards towards the floor so that the hands are pulled away from each other. You should now feel a stretch along the front and back of the arms along the pathways of the Heart Governor and Triple Heater Meridians. Hold for half a minute or so, breathing evenly, then breathe in and rise back up to a sitting position.

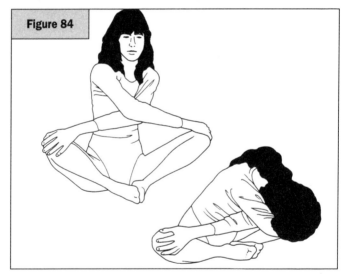

Figure 84

◆ Liver and Gall Bladder Meridian Stretch

Sitting on the floor, spread your legs as wide apart as they will comfortably go, while keeping them straight. Bending from the waist, reach down one leg with your hand as far as is comfortable, and bring the other arm over your head towards the same foot. Keep facing forwards rather than facing the leg, so that the side of your torso is stretched. Relax and breathe evenly. You should now be able to feel the pathways of the Liver and Gall Bladder Meridians being stretched on the inside and outside of the legs and in the side of the torso.

After holding for half a minute or more, breathe in as you sit up again, then breathe out and go down to the other leg. Again hold for at least half a minute while breathing evenly, then rise back up to a sitting position.

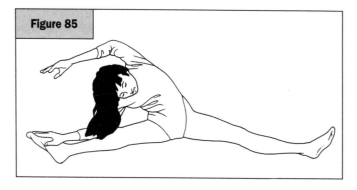

Figure 85

Now that you have finished the six exercises, lie down on your back with your arms to your sides for a few minutes. Relax, and tune into what is happening within your body. You may well be able to feel sensations of Energy moving around your body. When you feel ready, you can get up!

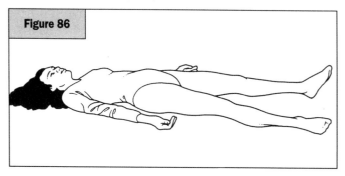

Figure 86

POSTSCRIPT

I hope that you have enjoyed this book, that the information has brought a new way of looking at your life and health, and that you have now given lots of Shiatsu to your friends. There is a lot of information in Part 3 that will take time for you to fully appreciate and put into practise, so you may well like to go back over this part of the book.

If you have enjoyed learning Shiatsu I encourage you to learn more by attending some classes with a qualified teacher. It is a great help in learning this very practical art to be taught at first hand. The Useful Addresses section at the end of this book has a list of the major schools running Shiatsu courses in Britain. If none of these are close to you, try contacting the Shiatsu Society which has a longer list of teachers. There are also a number of teachers and centres where you can find out more about food Energetics and its theraputic uses. The Community Health Foundation can supply a list of contacts throughout the country.

GLOSSARY

Anma A traditional form of massage used in Japan.

Astral body The subtle Energetic body associated with our emotions.

Aura The extension of the body's Energy beyond the physical body. Consists of a number of 'layers': the etheric, astral, mental and causal.

Barley malt A sweetener made from sprouted barley grains. Also called malt extract, it is used to sweeten cakes, cookies and other desserts, porridge, drinks, etc.

Causal body The subtle Energetic body associated with a person's soul or 'higher self'.

Chakra A wheel or centre of Energy within the Energetic body. There are seven main Chakras lying on the spiritual channel, and many more minor Chakras.

Energy Subtle Energy detectable by living organisms but not by mechanical instruments, to be distinguished from the Western idea of energy which is associated with matter. Called Ki in Japanese. For definition, see Ki.

Etheric body The densest subtle body closely associated with the physical functioning of the body.

Fu An Organ concerned with transforming food and drink into Energy for the body to use, and with excretion. Usually associated with a hollow organ, e.g. the Stomach.

Hara The Energetic centre in the lower abdomen.

Jitsu An excess of Energy.

Ki Ki is universal, found everywhere and in all things. It manifests in different ways to create physical forms and living organisms. In the human body it creates our physical, emotional, mental and spiritual being.

Kyo A deficiency in Energy.

Macrobiotics A reinterpretation of ancient Oriental philosophy and medicine, begun this century by George Ohsawa and now taught by Michio Kushi and other teachers. Emphasizes living in harmony with nature and universal laws, especially through eating an Energetically balanced diet.

Mental body The subtle Energetic body associated with the intellect, containing thoughtforms.

Meridian A channel of Energy travelling over the body's surface and internally through the organs of the body.

Miso A rich-tasting soya bean paste used for seasoning soups, stews and other vegetable dishes. Made by fermenting soya beans with grain and sea salt for over a year.

Moxibustion The application of heat to acupuncture points, for example by burning a small amount of dried mugwort on the skin.

Organ A group of functions including that of a physical organ, but also of other bodily functions, an emotion, tissue, sense organ and aspect of consciousness.

Spiritual Channel A channel of Energy running between the top of the head and the base of the torso. The seven main Chakras lie on the spiritual channel.

Subtle body An Energetic body overlying the physical body and extending beyond the physical body to form the aura.

Tsubo A point on the skin where the Energy flow of a Meridian or of the body can be beneficially affected. Tsubo is used to denote
a) an acupuncture point, and
b) any point on the body where Energy flow can be beneficially changed.

Yang Any phenomena or form in which Energy is primarily contracting or becoming more organised, e.g. animals, growth, work, introversion.

Yin Any phenomena or form in which Energy is primarily expanding or becoming more dispersed, e.g. decay, relaxation, expression.

Zang An Organ concerned with the storage of Energy, and usually associated with a solid organ, e.g. the Liver.

FURTHER READING

The Human Energetic Constitution

The Book of Do-in: Exercises for Physical and Spiritual Development, Michio Kushi. Japan Publications Inc., Tokyo, 1979.

Vibrational Medicine, Richard Gerber. Bear & Company, Santa Fe, 1988.

The Yellow Emperor's Classic of Internal Medicine, Ilza Veith. University of California Press, Los Angeles & London, 1966.

Shiatsu

The Book of Shiatsu, Saul Goodman. Avery, 1991.

Zen Shiatsu, Shizuto Masunaga and Wataru Ohashi. Japan Publications Inc., Tokyo, 1977.

Shiatsu Theory and Practice, C. Beresford-Cooke. Churchill Livingstone, 1996.

Food Energetics

Yin and Yang: A Practical Guide to Eating a Balanced and Healthy Diet, Oliver Cowmeadow. Cornish Connection, 1985.

Food For Thought: A New Look at Food and Behaviour, Saul Miller with Jo Anne Miller. Prentice-Hall Inc., N.J., 1985.

Food and Healing, Annemarie Colbin. Ballentine Books, 1986.

Oriental Diagnosis

Your Face Never Lies: An Introduction to Oriental Diagnosis, Michio Kushi. Avery Publishing Group Inc., 1983.

How To See Your Health: Book of Oriental Diagnosis, Michio Kushi. Japan Publications Inc., 1980.

Reading the Body, Wataru Ohashi, Arkana, 1991.

USEFUL ADDRESSES

For professional training courses in Shiatsu in the UK contact:

The Devon School of Shiatsu
The Coach House, Buckyette Farm, Littlehempston, Totnes,
Devon TQ9 6ND
Tel: 01803 762593
www.devonshiatsu.co.uk
email: info@devonshiatsu.co.uk

To find a Shiatsu therapist or Shiatsu school in your area
contact one of the following:

The Shiatsu Society (UK)
Eastlands Court, St Peters Road, Rugby CV21 3QP
Tel: 0845 130 4560
www.shiatsu.org
email: admin@shiatsu.org

American Organisation for Bodywork Therapies
1010 Haddon Field, Berlin Road, Suite 408, Voorhees,
New Jersey 08043
Tel: 00856 782 1616

Shiatsu Therapy Association of Australia
PO Box 598, Belgrave, Victoria 3160
Tel: 0061 039 457 5834

INDEX

The Indexer has aimed to use Capital letters to represent Oriental concepts (e.g. Energy, Kidney) reflecting usage in the text (see Note on p.4). Any accidental lapses in this method are entirely the responsibility of the Indexer.

A

B

arms, 149
face, 149, 150
intercostal, 151
shoulders, 149
nose, 22, 151
bleeding, 155
congestion, 150, 151
numbness, 151

O

Ocean of Blood Tsubo, 150
Ocean of Ki Tsubo, 155
operations, 46
Organs, 24-6, 169
Orgone Energy, 8 *and see* Energy
osteoarthritis, 126
Outer Gate Tsubo, 153
overweight, 150 *and see* fat

P

pain, 9, 99, 101
abdomen, 150, 155
ankles, 150, 154
arms, 149
back, 128-9, 130-1, 151, 152, 154
calves, 154
chest, 149, 152, 155
elbow, 149
eyes, 152
feet, 152
knees, 156
menstrual, 150
neck, 154
ribs, 154
shoulders, 149, 151, 153, 154
stomach, 150
wrists, 149
and see aches
Palace of Hearing Tsubo, 151
palpitations, 153, 155
pancreas, 22, 25, 124-5, 130, 133, 137, 139
paralysis, 149, 150, 151
Pericardium Organ *see* Heart Governor Organ
personal power, 22, 137
pharyngitis, 149
piles, 149, 155
Pillar of Heaven Tsubo, 151
pineal gland, 22
pituitary gland, 22
Place of Anxiety Tsubo, 153
pneumonia, 151 *and see* lungs
Prana, 8 and see Energy
pregnancy, 45, 46, 131, 145, 152 *and see* childbirth

throat, 22
   soreness, 149, 150, 155
Throat Chakra, 22
thymus, 22
thyroid, 22
tinnitis, 151, 153
tiredness, 47
   eyes, 151
   legs, 150, 152
   and see exhaustion; fatigue
toes, 135
tonsillitis, 149
toothache, 149, 150, 153
Top of Shoulder Tsubo, 153
Transportation Place Tsubo, 152
treatments
   adapting, 94-5, 100-1
   discomfort/pain during, 99
   effects of, 46-50
   and emotion, 45, 49
   preparation for, 42-4
   principles of, 65
   resistance to, 138
   sequence, 66-7
   when not to give, 44-6
   and wholeness, 141
   and see Shiatsu
Triple Burner *see* Triple Heater Organ
Triple Heater Meridian
   stretch exercise, 164
   Tsubos, 146-8, 153
Triple Heater Organ, 26
Tsubos, 8, 27, 31, 169
   English names, 149-56
   how to use, 144-5, 149-56
   location, 143, 146-8, 149-56
   and Meridians, 142
   numbers, 149-56
   and Shiatsu, 143
   uses of, 143, 149-56
tumours, 112
turning over, 74

U

ulcers, stomach, 155
unconscious, 124
unconsciousness, 149, 150
understanding, 22
urinary problems, 152, 154
uterine bleeding, 151

V

Vagus nerve, 22
vertebrae, misaligned, 129, 131 *and see* back
vertigo, 153 *and see* dizziness
vitality, 22, 25, 152
    and diet, 132
    lack of, 154
vocal chords, 22
vomiting, 153

W

weakness, 151
    legs, 9, 151, 154
weight, how much to give, 61-2
Welcome Fragrance Tsubo, 149
Whole Bone Tsubo, 153
will power, 25, 151, 155
Wind Palace Tsubo, 155
Windy Pond Tsubo, 153
withdrawn nature, 128
wrists, 140, 149
writer's cramp, 153

X

Xiyan Knee Eyes Tsubo, 156

Y

Yang, 169
    foods, 111, 124, 126
Yang Hill Spring Tsubo, 154
Yin, 169
    foods, 111-12, 125, 132
Yin and Yang, 103-5, 169
    and diet, 109-12, 118, 132
    and food, 106-9
    and see balance
Yintang Seal Hall Tsubo, 156

Z

Zang, 24-6, 169